# A Valiant Battle:
## A Journey with Schizophrenia

Wendel L. Miser

with

James S. Miser, MD

For more information about this title or to order other books
and/or electronic media, contact the publisher:

Atkins & Greenspan Publishing
TwoSistersWriting.com
18530 Mack Avenue, Suite 166
Grosse Pointe Farms, MI 48236

ISBN:
978-1-956879-18-6 (Hardcover)
978-1-956879-19-3 (Paperback)
978-1-956879-20-9 (eBook)

Printed in the United States of America

All the stories in this work are true.

Cover: The Miser Family. Wendel Miser painted the picture
on the front cover as a boy. The painting on the back cover
has been in the Miser family for many years.

Author photos: The Miser Family Collection.

All Bible citations are from the King James Version published in
1611 by the American Bible Society in New York and are in the public domain.

Cover and Interior design: Van-garde Imagery

# Dedication

THIS BOOK IS DEDICATED to my wife, Mary, for her love and support. Words are inadequate to describe her unwavering courage and compassion in confronting the disease that has changed our lives and has affected our relationship forever. She has remained steadfastly at my side and has allowed me to heal, even though the process of healing has often been painfully slow.

The book is also dedicated to my psychiatrist, Dr. John Maloney, for his continuous commitment and care—he steered my spirit back to me; and to my brother, Jim, for his encouragement and support in bringing me closer to the Lord.

# Contents

Dedication . . . . . . . . . . . . . . . . . . . . iii

Foreword . . . . . . . . . . . . . . . . . . . .vii

Introduction . . . . . . . . . . . . . . . . . . ix

**Section 1**    **Journey to Despair**

Chapter 1    The Break — June 1978. . . . . . . . . . . . . 3

Chapter 2    The Four Days Before . . . . . . . . . . . . . .11

**Section 2**    **The Journey Before**

Chapter 3    My Family and The Early Years . . . . . . . . .17

Chapter 4    Andy . . . . . . . . . . . . . . . . . . . . . .19

Chapter 5    Mary . . . . . . . . . . . . . . . . . . . . . .27

Chapter 6    First Year at The Environmental
Protection Agency. . . . . . . . . . . . . . . .35

**Section 3**    **Journey Out of Loneliness**

Chapter 7    The Loneliness . . . . . . . . . . . . . . . . .43

Chapter 8    The Struggle to Stay Well . . . . . . . . . . .47

Chapter 9    The Family's Response . . . . . . . . . . . .49

Chapter 10    The Conversion . . . . . . . . . . . . . . . . .59

**Section 4**      **Journey to Joy**

Chapter 11    The Beginning of The Journey. . . . . . . . .67

Chapter 12    The Journey Continues — 1. . . . . . . . . .77

Chapter 13    The Journey Continues — 2. . . . . . . . . .93

**Section 5**      **The Joy**

Chapter 14    The Experience of Joy . . . . . . . . . . . . 103

                   Afterword. . . . . . . . . . . . . . . . 127

                   God's Reassurance. . . . . . . . . . . . 133

                   Acknowledgments. . . . . . . . . . . . 135

                   Bibliography . . . . . . . . . . . . . . . 137

                   Author Bio . . . . . . . . . . . . . . . . 139

                   Endnotes . . . . . . . . . . . . . . . . 145

# Foreword

MR. WENDEL MISER HAS been known to me since 1978, a year after he came to Washington, D.C. from Connecticut to work for the federal government. We met on the locked psychiatric ward of the George Washington University Hospital where he had recently been admitted. As his assigned psychiatrist, the staff and I prepared his treatment plan, which included medication and seclusion from other patients in order to restore his level of functioning.

He did improve and was discharged to outpatient care. There was some initial reluctance to take medication due to side effects, which resulted in relapse and return to the inpatient unit on a couple of occasions.

Mr. Miser has been my longest continually active patient since 1978. We have consistently met for psychotherapy with medication management with various durations between appointments. Most recently, we have been meeting through telemedicine due to the Covid pandemic about every three to four weeks. Early in the therapy, there was some group therapy and occasional joint meetings with his wife.

During the course of therapy, Mr. Miser has shown initiative to broaden his experiences. He began journaling his thoughts that have resulted in this and two other potential books. He began exploring religious thought more seriously and became active in his church to include becoming an elder and giving presentations to the congregation. He became active in singing and performed with multiple choruses in D.C. and Virginia. He was able to retire from the federal agency he started with after obtaining several awards. He was fortunate to have the support of his family, the church, and his choirs to which he contributed.

This book is about the journey of a man initially diagnosed with a serious mental illness over four decades ago and his determination and resilience to work through it. It is his intent to share this with you so that you may benefit from his experience.

John R. Maloney, MD<br>
McLean, Virginia

# Introduction

THIS IS A STORY of hope and of overcoming an illness that has profoundly affected the course of my life. Some of the story is difficult to read, but the destination of the journey is one of great joy. Many individuals in our world today are afflicted with psychiatric illness. When confronted with someone who has such a challenging condition, most of us shrink back out of fear and ignorance. By responding this way, however, the isolation of the sufferer becomes even more profound.

Many people have had a significantly positive impact on my life and have helped me on my journey of overcoming schizophrenia. Since the onset of the disease, they have helped to nurture me back to health and productivity. Their courage to confront my illness was a tremendous help in my healing. Many have told me about Jesus, by sharing their own stories and their relationship to Him. This story is also about them, those individuals who supported, embraced and loved me as I was so I could heal. They have been a blessing to me.

As I look back over time and remember this road to health, I am thankful for the gifts of good doctors and the medical treatments they use to thwart debilitating psychiatric illness. Several years ago, my psychiatrist Dr. John R. Maloney quoted Dr. William Osler, a famous physician: "If you want to live a long life, contract a chronic disease and take care of it."

Dr. Maloney has allowed me to do this with his support. Jim, a doctor dedicated to caring for children with cancer, has approached me as a brother in the deepest sense. He has embraced me with an unconditional love, the love from God that is available to everyone.

With schizophrenia, there is unavoidable stigma. As the years have passed with Dr. Maloney's care, I have faced a barrage of confused emotions. A basic feeling of mine for so long was that I just didn't fit in. Normalcy, sensitivity, integrity, balance, and compassion are feelings for which I have yearned. Often, I have been confused about relationships and circumstances. With Dr. Maloney's care and love from family and friends, as Dr. Maloney puts it, I am now free to be myself. That being so, I wear this disease as a multi-layered set of clothes never quite fitting as it should. After all is said and done, however, I have come to feel very special.

I realize there are people who will never understand schizophrenia nor accept the person who is saddled with it. They are the ones who will have a position about me, the schizophrenic. They will try to get used to me, to put up with me, or to even stay away from me. This position does not allow me to feel free or special.

Schizophrenia is an illness that I have. It is not who I am. Treating me as a diagnosis without getting to know me as a person traps me and hurts me deeply. An approach to me based on acceptance results in feelings of meaning and love. Family, friends, and colleagues who have approached me as I am, find me. With their love and support, I can more easily give back.

I have come to appreciate the story of the 10 lepers and the one who returned to thank Jesus. As it was in the days of Jesus when leprosy was horribly misunderstood, it is today with schizophrenia.

Struggling with this diagnosis, I, too, have gone to Jesus truly thankful for the healing I have received.

A passage from the King James Version of the Bible in Luke 17:11-19 is very special to me:

> *11 And it came to pass, as he went to Jerusalem, that he passed through the midst of Samaria and Galilee.*
>
> *12 And as he entered into a certain village, there met him ten men that were lepers, which stood afar off:*
>
> *13 And they lifted up their voices, and said, Jesus, Master, have mercy on us.*
>
> *14 And when he saw them, he said unto them, Go show yourselves unto the priests. And it came to pass, that, as they went, they were cleansed.*
>
> *15 And one of them, when he saw that he was healed, turned back, and with a loud voice glorified God,*
>
> *16 And fell down on his face at his feet, giving him thanks: and he was a Samaritan.*
>
> *17 And Jesus answering said, Were there not ten cleansed? but where are the nine?*
>
> *18 There are not found that returned to give glory to God, save this stranger.*
>
> *19 And he said unto him, Arise, go thy way: thy faith hath made thee whole.*[1]

As I came to understand Jesus' teachings, it became clear that I was to be separate from the ways of the world, but remain in the world. I am God's adopted son. The joy I find in Jesus is profound, a joy that is life-sustaining, evidenced by the hope, love, and grace embodied in Jesus' sacrifice for us all. My heart sings of a new freedom given to me by His loving act on the cross that released me from years of imprisonment by a disease marked by directionless living. My life now has purpose and meaning, made possible by my discovery and acceptance of Jesus as Lord of my life. Early in my journey, Jim shared this scripture from Romans 8:38-39 with me:

> *38 For I am persuaded, that neither death, nor life, nor angels, nor principalities, nor powers, nor things present, nor things to come,*

> *39 Nor height, nor depth, nor any other creature, shall be able to separate us from the love of God, which is in Christ Jesus our Lord.*[2]

I now know that I can never be separated from the love of God.

## Section 1
# Journey to Despair

*"The thing that preserves a man from panic is his relationship to God; if he is only related to himself and to his own courage, there may come a moment when his courage gives out."*

The Complete Works of Oswald Chambers
Discovery House, *2000*[1]

---

# Chapter 1

# The Break — June 1978

I CURLED UP IN a ball in the dining room on the floor, afraid. Afraid to go anywhere. Afraid to do anything. Curled up, I closed the world out, trapping myself inside my own prison without bars that kept me confined. Time passed—minutes, hours, or days, I was not sure. Frozen in time, I didn't know what to do or where to turn. I had no comfort zone. My reality had suddenly changed, its details now sharp and bright, and beyond real.

As I had gone to bed the night before, panic had set in. Looking at the clock on the nightstand, the second hand had stood still, paralyzing me in time. I was terrified, caught in a moment of time, disconnected from the world, and distant from Mary, my wife, and all that was around me.

Sleep came, but it was intermittent and disturbed. Neither my body nor my mind could rest. In the morning, I awoke scared. I went to the kitchen, terrified by my detachment from the reality of the simplest kitchen items: the window, the table, and a bowl of fruit.

In a frenzy, I unplugged all the appliances, big and small, to protect myself from the power in the walls that I feared. Turning back to the dining room, away from the frightening things I had confronted in the kitchen, I sank to the floor.

Later, driven to the hospital emergency room by close friends, I spit an egg salad sandwich out the window of the car that was no longer edible to me. In the waiting room, I felt imprisoned. No one came. No one listened. No one paid attention. No one cared.

"This is all bullshit!" I screamed over and over to an uncaring world as I waited.

The staff and other patients whispered amongst themselves and looked on in horror.

Restrained by security, I was taken to a Quiet Room in the psychiatric ward, where behind a locked door, I screamed, "Where are you, Mary? Get me out of here!"

I was so alone, so afraid, forced to be confined with only a radiator and a urinal I didn't use. I relieved myself in the corner. The hot radiator singed my hand.

"There is an atomic bomb in the radiator," I screamed, warning the world of its impending doom. I recoiled from the danger in anxiety and nervous fear.

The world was in my face. Everything was in my face. And yet I was so alone. There was no space for Mary. No space for Andy, my twin brother. My consciousness was streaming faster than I could comprehend. The details of my reality overwhelmed my senses with sharpness, intensity, and speed.

And then I slowly drifted into the oblivion of a drug-induced haze caused by medications prescribed to bring me back to reality from my psychotic break.

Schizophrenia.

*Here's how it happened in the words of my loved ones.*

## My Brother, Jim

*I couldn't breathe. I felt like I had just been kicked in the stomach. I could not speak. Mary was on the phone: "Jim, Wendel is in the hospital; he has had a psychotic break."*

*Standing in the corner of the kitchen of our Ohio farmhouse, I slumped against the wall, barely able to stay on my feet. Earlier in my career, I had spent time with psychiatric patients: rows of individuals in ward after ward; repetitive behaviors; no apparent meaningful interactions with those around them; some with no movement at all; some obviously afraid of everything in their surroundings.*

*These images had shocked me at the time. They were also the images that came to my mind now as I spoke to Mary on the phone. Was this really touching Wendel's life and the life of his wife, Mary? Was this really touching our lives as a family? Would he be hospitalized forever—institutionalized, unable to relate to me? Were there good drugs to treat whatever he had? And what would the side effects be? These were my initial frantic thoughts.*

*The weight on my chest and on my heart was heavy, and I sobbed. 'What can I do?' I thought.*

*I said to my wife, "Angela, we need to go to Washington to be with Mary and the family. Wendel has had a psychotic break." And then I made arrangements to come to Washington, D.C. to be with my brother and my family, not knowing whether I would ever be able to communicate with him again.*

### My Sister, Emily

*Mom called: "Something has happened to Wendel. He has had a nervous breakdown."*

*I didn't understand at all. What was happening to Wendel? What was happening to our family? There didn't seem to be clear language to talk about it. I had recently moved to Boston and struggled to find my first job. I felt unsettled and uncertain professionally. And now this shock.*

*I travelled to Washington with my parents to see Wendel in the hospital. It was awkward and strange. I wanted to understand what was happening to Wendel and I didn't want Mary to be upset or angry. I had no idea how to help and my parents didn't seem to be very helpful, either. I have dim memories of the time after that.*

### My Brother, Andy

*I was stunned and shocked, completely unprepared. It took me by complete surprise.*

*I got a call at home in Hartford that Wendel had landed in the psychiatric hospital at George Washington University, having suffered an acute mental breakdown. After talking to my wife, Martha, and my parents, trying to figure out what I was going to do, I made arrangements to fly with my mother to Washington, D.C., to stay with Mary and to see Wendel in the hospital. My life was all of a sudden upside-down and topsy-turvy. I was terrified.*

*After Mom and I arrived in Washington, we went with Mary to the hospital to see Wendel, who was in a room by himself. We waited for what seemed hours before we had a chance to see him.*

*Wendel was still drowsy when I came into the room. He was lying on a drab mattress on the floor, curled up and very drowsy. His good ear was down in the pillow and his deaf left ear up to the world, shutting out the sounds of the experience around him; however, he was somehow aware that I was with him, even though the medications being used to stabilize him compelled him to sleep.*

*There was no other furniture in the room, except a chair. Sitting on the edge of the bed, I touched his shoulder and asked him to roll over to hear me. He recognized me and smiled, but then turned away, wanting to sleep. I stayed with him for a while. We spoke very little.*

*After a brief time together, Wendel walked me to the door that let me out and closed him in to the barrenness of a locked reality. As I left, we peered at each other through the little window in the confining door. I was on one side in the doorway, he on the other. I looked at him and gave him the universal OK sign.*

*"Wendel, it will be OK," I said through the window glass. Our eyes locked together. I will never forget the extraordinary moment, a thread connecting us. I had no real certainty at all that it was ever going to be OK.*

*Although declaring through the window that he would recover, in the loneliness of my heart, I was terrified: not sure of the path forward, not sure of his healing, not sure that the illness would not permanently alter our relationship, not sure that we would be together again, not sure whether I would be OK. In the weeks that followed after returning home, I continued to wonder if Wendel would ever recover, if he would ever be happy again. I wondered if I would ever really be happy again.*

## My Wife, Mary

*Wendel and I were married in Connecticut nearly six years prior to his psychotic break. Following our wedding, we headed to the University of Illinois at Urbana-Champaign, where Wendel began a graduate program and earned a Master's degree in Zoology. After finishing the graduate program, we returned to Connecticut for a short time until he was hired by the U.S. Environmental Protection Agency in Washington, D.C. It was an exciting and happy time. We had grown into a strong and independent couple. And then, things changed.*

*I was very frightened. Afraid of losing my marriage. Afraid of losing Wendel, my husband, my lover, my companion, my friend... forever. I didn't know where to turn, so I called Andy's father-in-law, a physician. Recognizing the seriousness of Wendel's condition, he advised me to take him to George Washington University immediately. I was very grateful for his concern and advice that I quickly followed.*

*Who were these doctors and nurses who seemed to think they knew my husband? How was any of this going to bring Wendel out of his psychotic stupor? Would he ever be discharged from the hospital? Why was this happening? What exactly was happening?*

*There was nothing in my realm of experience to prepare*

me for Wendel's break. I could only watch as he became increasingly fearful, restless, and finally, so out of touch with reality that by Sunday, it was difficult to recognize the same person I had known and loved on Friday.

Dr. John Maloney happened to be the psychiatrist on call on the weekend of Wendel's first episode. My initial interaction with Dr. Maloney was not pleasant. I was upset and he needed me to encourage Wendel to sign the insurance forms. I scoffed and said, "It's always about money, isn't it."

I was immediately sorry I had said that, but I could not contain my distress at losing my healthy husband. I was going to need help and gathered enough presence of mind to know that Dr. Maloney was likely our "get out of jail card" if I even dared to hope for any kind of recovery for Wendel. But what were all these terms, these medications?

### In the Hospital

Later in the hospitalization, I intensely studied a chalkboard with a list of hundreds of fun things to do in Washington, D.C. But I felt completely divorced from the concept of doing anything for enjoyment. Nor could I convince myself that I was going to be OK, or even understand what that meant. Little did I know that the journey to that place of being OK would be so long and difficult.

My life was shattered.

Chapter 2

# The Four Days Before

THE FOUR DAYS BEFORE had been very stressful and difficult. I was unable to concentrate and was filled with anxiety. Thursday afternoon after work, I was expected to participate in a softball game on one of the many public fields in Washington, D.C. As I ventured off to the diamond near Haines Point with a group of friends, I became gradually detached from their energy and conversation. Although I loved baseball, during the game I was distracted and entranced by a group of children playing nearby, so much so that I completely lost track of the progression and score of the game. I was not engaged in playing the game.

"Get in the game, Wendel," admonished a teammate.

I was separated from the team and its attempt to win. I lost track of time and became disoriented about where I was. At the end of the game, confused, I had asked one of my teammates,

"Can I have a ride home?"

"How far do you need to go?" he asked.

Another worried friend directed, "He needs to go home."

Not realizing the depth of my confusion, my teammate let me off at a telephone booth at an exit along the Interstate 395 corridor.

Alone, I struggled to find my telephone number to call Mary. Not knowing where I was, I asked a complete stranger for help. He gave me my location, which I confusedly relayed to Mary, who came and rescued me. She questioned me about my day and why I had taken two white pills that someone had given me, confirmed later to be only aspirin provided to me by a friend for a headache. When Mary presented me a small gift of a framed set of butterflies she had coincidentally purchased for me that day, I cried, but didn't know why.

I told her, "I think I had a nervous breakdown today."

Mary became increasingly concerned about the disorientation I was exhibiting, but was unsure whether I needed medical care at that time.

## Mary

*A few weeks before, I had read an article in a magazine about PCP (phencyclidine) and its increasing popularity in the United States. I had no experience and little knowledge of the use of "recreational drugs," but I was fascinated by the ease with which young people were latching on to "angel dust" in the Washington, D.C. area. The effects that even a small dose of the drug had on some people seemed appalling to me. Among the side effects were paranoia, slurred speech, and changes in normal behavior.*

*Wendel was paranoid. At times he would not speak at all or, when he did speak, it was nonsense. His behavior was anything but normal. Initially, I was concerned about the two white pills he had been given. I could not verbalize that perhaps he had fallen prey to this PCP that had become so popular. He had told me that someone at work that day had given him two small white pills. (I learned years later that the two white pills he had been given were merely aspirin because he complained of a headache.)*

*Further, Wendel had never abused any drug, including PCP. Worse than this fear, Wendel had lost touch with reality. He was by himself, in a world of confusion, suspicion, and mistrust. Mentally, he seemed to be drifting somewhere very far off. I felt that he was shutting me out, but realized early on that he did not want to take me to that dark place with him. To my horror, I had to accept that Wendel was mentally ill.*

*On lunch hour that day, I had gone to a nearby gift shop where I had found some butterflies mounted and nicely framed. I knew Wendel would like the gift. As a biologist, he was always fascinated with butterflies, and I was delighted with my purchase. When I gave him the butterflies that evening, however, he began to cry. Initially, I was touched that he should be so moved by the gift, but I soon realized that his tears were not a reaction to the gift. He told me that he had had a nervous breakdown that day.*

*My immediate reaction was one of doubt and skepticism, bordering on cynicism. I was quite certain that I would be the champion without question, had anyone looked at the two of us and asked, "Which of these two people is about to have a nervous breakdown?"*

*The next few days threw my mind, my body, my emotions, and my faith into a whirlwind of doubt, fear, anger, and heartbreak. What had happened, seemingly overnight?*

## That Night

I was confused and wasn't eating well. That night I was unable to sleep. Concerned about me, the next morning Mary wrestled with whether she should go to work. Together we rationalized that I was just over-tired and she went to work while I stayed home.

Later that morning, very disoriented, I appeared at our neighbor's front door in my underwear. They called Mary, who came home from work and took me to the hospital for evaluation. Now knowing that I was not just over-tired, she feared that she was losing hold of the husband whom she loved. At the Emergency Room, the psychiatric nurse, recognizing that I was having difficulties, instructed Mary that she should bring me back if I became more disoriented.

The next two nights, I could neither keep my eyes closed nor sleep. By then, my break from reality was complete. No one and nothing made sense.

At the time of the sudden onset of my illness, I was 28 years old and had been happily married to Mary, my lover, my confidant, and my closest friend, for six years.

Section 2

# The Journey Before

# Chapter 3
# My Family and The Early Years

UNTIL MY BREAK, MY life had followed a normal and happy path. I had grown up in a typical family. I have an older brother, a younger sister, and a twin brother. We did things together as a family: church, vacations, and family gatherings.

One of my earliest memories of church and Sunday school with family was being introduced to Psalm 100, a psalm of God's goodness and our response of joy, thanksgiving, and praise to Him. I remember being struck at that early age by these written words of comfort: "It is He that hath made us, and not we ourselves." At that early age, I began to know His importance in my life.

My father was a mathematician and professional in the discipline of Operations Research, for which he was an editor. Dad always wore a bow tie and carried a pocket watch and a handkerchief. When I would come down to breakfast in the early morning, Dad would be reading the funny papers with his bow tie hanging on each side of his neck.

Dad and I shared a number of passions: music, baseball, and singing. We enjoyed being together and I was certain of his love for me. He always made me feel special. His integrity and honesty in his professional life were an example for me in mine.

Dad shared his love of classical music with me. When I was 10, he introduced me to D'Indy's *Symphony on a French Mountain Air,* which became a favorite for me. Through junior high school, Mom and Dad would play piano duets in the living room, the melodious sounds of which would carry through the floor of my room above as I studied.

My mother was trained in child development and was at home during all of my childhood. She was an unconditional lover of people, a character builder, and a moral compass. When in my searching I would go to her, she would teach a little, love a lot, and bless much along the way. I now realize that her love for me was based on the hope that is in the Lord's promise of forgiveness. She would say to me that the love you give is the only love you keep.

Chapter 4

# Andy

MY TWIN BROTHER, ANDY, and I were born one minute apart on Saturday, April 22, 1950.

Andy was always easy to love. He was always with me. I was like him and he was like me. Life was wide-eyed for the two of us then. Andy made me aware of a poem by Edwin Markham, a 19th and 20th century Disciples of Christ poet:

> *"He drew a circle that shut me out—*
> *Heretic, rebel, a thing to flout.*
> *But Love and I had the wit to win*
> *And we drew a circle that took him in!"* [3]

> — Edwin Markham
> Chalice Hymnal, 1995

I understood this poem as representing Andy's love for me. Deaf in my left ear, I thought more than once that because I had difficulty hearing, that he might have felt that I shut him out of situations and conversations. I imagined then that he, on the other hand, drew a circle that took me in.

## Andy

*Wendy was born first, I was born second, so he is always going to be older and I am always going to be younger by one minute. We were born into the world as twins. A tandem. A duo. A pair. We were born Andrew and Wendel, alias, Andy and Wendy. Not only were there two of us, but we were identical. The same. We came into the world as identical twins. Being twins, each of us was already and always defined in relationship to the other one. That's just the way it was.*

*It was not, "Hey, look at Andy, isn't he handsome?" Or, "Wow, look at Wendy, isn't he good looking?"*

*It was always, "Hey, look at the twins, aren't they cute?" Our unique individual selves were secondary to our "twin-ness."*

*My childhood was all about Wendel and me, at least that is how I remember it. From the earliest times, he and I had joint ownership of each of our lives, inseparable in our cribs and later in our shared room. Growing up, Wendy was always there. I'd wake up each morning and there was Wendy.*

## Life with My Twin Brother

My one big moment when I took things into my own hands, however, was when I became the proud owner of Big Bearie, a very special, large maroon stuffed bear, after the successful trade of my brothers' train set to a friend down the street. Andy was not pleased with my bargaining alone. Jim didn't seem to care. And I had Big Bearie. I still do, stuffed away somewhere in a closet.

Andy was my constant partner, with our toy tool sets imitating

Dad, in moments alone together in a world of make-believe or on our Schwinn bicycles, together pedaling newspapers around a double-sized route. After we collected muddy redeemable bottles together under the local stadium, the grocery store manager on receiving our dirty collection made it very clear after giving us $2.00 for our first haul, "Never again!"

## Andy

*Before we turned 10 years old, we were always "the twins." Being twins meant having a built-in playmate all the time. We were happy playing all day together and sharing everything. We were not really competitive with each other. We played together and made sure that we both got the same things.*

*Fairness was important. Wendy and I had a rule that if we were getting a drink of lemonade or some chocolate cake, one of us would pour the lemonade or cut the cake and other one of us would be able to choose first. That always ensured that each of us got the same amount of whatever we were eating or drinking. It was the twin thing.*

*Growing up, Mom often dressed us alike. We would go off to junior high school with matching green bookbags over our shoulders and matching outfits. Later, wanting to be different in high school, we would discover at breakfast that we had dressed identically, forcing one of us to change before leaving for school.*

*Being twins means having other people always look surprised by our likeness and having people unable to tell us apart. I was often called Wendy. Wendy was often called*

*Andy. That was fun much of the time as we enjoyed fooling people.*

*Being a twin, I often felt special, different, not like other people. "Twin-ness" was always in the background of our lives and something I knew was there, but paid attention to only when others pointed it out. It was just normal to have a brother who looked like me, talked like me, and acted like me.*

*We did celebrate our differences, though. I'm left-handed and he's right-handed and what we loved to tell people was that everything I did right, he did left. For instance, I batted right and threw left, and he batted left and threw right.*

*We shared a bedroom while growing up. I had my bed and he had his. Everything else, we shared. Whenever he and I would receive gifts, for instance on our birthday or on Christmas morning, we got the same thing. Maybe they were a different color, but we got the same pair of pants, the same shirt, the same cowboy hat, and the same six-shooter with a holster.*

*We loved to watch the Lone Ranger on television and then go outside and play cowboys and Indians. We were always on the same side—the good guys. We loved to play in the woods together. I remember we would cross the small brook at the bottom of a long, overgrown roadway that went down a slope into the woods surrounding our home. More than once, one of us would fall into the brook and would have to trudge home to change into dry clothes.*

*One winter, Wendy and I made a path through freshly fallen snow in the woods with our snow shovels. We would also do that with leaves. We loved to make paths and we would walk through the woods following the paths we had created.*

*We would also go out into the woods and explore for lost treasure. We found an old truck, rusted and hidden by the overgrowth. We did not dare to get in or to explore too closely. There was something scary about that vehicle. What was it doing out in the woods? How did it get there? Our imaginations would run wild and we would make stories about the bad guy who had left it there. We were always on some kind of adventure that we had created together in our imaginations.*

## Our Adventures

Andy was my partner in tennis, in whiffle ball, in a singing tour around New England, in tossing eggs and snowballs (we got into a little trouble), in collecting coins, and in pillow fights. The pillow fights became especially vigorous when our cousins arrived, resulting in a baptism of feathers about which our parents were not pleased.

Andy and I started collecting United States coins just after Mom and Dad moved to Lincoln, Massachusetts in 1960. We were both struck by the rich revolutionary and literary history of the neighboring towns of Concord and Lexington that we both remember visiting by bicycle past Walden Pond on a regular basis.

As part of our adventures, we explored in and around the battleground areas by foot, whether it was at the Old North Bridge in Concord or the Lexington Green. We would often frequent a small coin shop in Concord's main square and quickly became fascinated with coins to collect. Both old and new coins were intriguing—old coins for their imagined past and new coins for their beautiful luster and minted perfection.

We started with what we could afford, exchanging pocket change for a collectible coin. At the time, many of the coins had silver content: Washington quarters, Mercury head dimes, and Roosevelt dimes, to name a few. We saved our money to buy them. Shortly after President John F. Kennedy was assassinated, the Kennedy half dollar become an instant collectible. Mom had quite a few liberty dollars that she gave to us for safekeeping. Our favorite coin was the Mercury head dime, not by an agreed-upon standard, but to our surprise, out of our common interest.

What made coin collecting fun was periodically quoting their possible worth from the "red" book that gave prices in connection with the condition of the coins—excellent, good, and fair. We never intended to become "wealthy" collecting coins—we did it for the sheer fun of doing it together. It connected us to history and the world around us and to each other.

We were always close and occasionally substituted for each other, much to the consternation of our teachers. Although I occasionally compared my achievement to Andy's, I was never particularly aware of an academic competition between the two of us while in junior or senior high school.

We did, however, enjoy some competitive activities. Once, we were opposing pitchers in a Little League game, the Pirates versus the Giants. Andy and I each pitched the whole game for our respective teams. Dad called balls and strikes, an intimidating presence for both of us. In the seventh and last inning, my center fielder dropped the ball and my team lost. It hurt badly.

## Andy

*I can remember Wendy and me watching Dad working on his model railroad trains, being there at the front door when Dad brought home our first television and listening to Leroy Anderson on the phonograph in Dad's office off the kitchen.*

*I remember when Dad showed us how he played the trumpet. I was so upset on Christmas when Wendy got a trumpet and I got a guitar. We never did learn to play either one of them.*

## Companionship

Andy's sense of humor put me at ease in social situations and being together in most settings was as natural as the world revolving on its axis. His companionship was what I cherished the most. After high school, we took separate paths, coming back together for college vacations and family get-togethers. The separation was difficult.

Chapter 5

# Mary

I MET MARY ON a double date with Andy in the backyard of Andy's girlfriend. It was love at first sight and she has remained the only girl in my life throughout high school, college, and to the present. Her experience growing up in a large family with six brothers and two sisters would be of great value to her as she partnered in caring for me.

May Yay, her pronunciation of "Mary" and her nickname as a young child, is the seventh child of two seventh children who was born on the fifth day of the fifth month in 1950.

Living beside the Farmington River in Unionville, Connecticut as a child, she experienced its flooding in 1955 when her family lost their home and depended on the Red Cross in its aftermath. In the years that followed, her father built another home at the foot of Taine Mountain in Unionville at a higher elevation after the flood subsided. I am sure her sense of perseverance, which I have come to know so well, was already developing at that time.

A week after our wedding in September 1972, Mary and I began our life together in Urbana, Illinois, where I started my graduate work at the University of Illinois in the Departments of Civil Engineering and Zoology.

Pop, my maternal grandfather, a professor of Agricultural

Engineering at the University of Illinois in Urbana, died in October of that year and I have always thought it would have been very special to have gotten to know him better. When my uncle Bill put Pop's house up to be sold, he asked the two of us if we would like to live there during the time it was on the market. Bill believed that, in addition to helping us out, it would be better to have the house occupied while he was trying to sell it. A win-win situation.

We took him up on his offer and lived there for six months. We had very little furniture and in such a big house, we could not get rid of the echo on all levels, due to the emptiness. We made our bedroom in Pop's study on the first floor off the living room. We didn't use the top floor because of the lack of heat.

In the evenings, we would listen to *Mystery Theater*, a radio program starring E. G. Marshall. We would sit in the large living room with no fire and the lights turned off and listen to the tale that he would spin. In the pitch black, we would huddle together, being spooked.

After a buyer was found, we spent the summer in the adjacent barn, fully finished as an apartment. Later that summer, Grandfather Miser was traveling through the area by car and stopped to see us there. The time spent at Perkins Road has become a wonderful memory for both of us and was great for our marriage. We remained emotionally close to both of our families, despite being apart 24 hours by car. Mary did miss her family in Connecticut.

In 1975, after completing my Master's Thesis, I had to defend my conclusions by oral examination. Shortly before I graduated, a team of five professors and I met for the challenge. They were on one side of the table, I on the other. I was asked 10 questions, nine of which I answered successfully in the time allowed. When it came to the last question, I was not immediately forthcoming. I hemmed and hawed, and after consideration, I told the group that I had no answer.

The Chairman of the panel said, "That's okay, Wendel, neither do we."

At that moment, I felt incredibly relieved, but realized at the same time that if I had tried to give an answer, I may not have passed the oral exam. The experience taught me that an honest "I do not know" to a question about a subject I knew little about was a legitimate and good answer to give.

One of the most precious memories I have of Mary is that every Christmas she would reflect on the Christmas story in Luke 2:8-14:

*8 And there were in the same country shepherds abiding in the field, keeping watch over their flock by night.*

*9 And, lo, the angel of the Lord came upon them, and the glory of the Lord shone round about them: and they were sore afraid.*

*10 And the angel said unto them, Fear not: for, behold, I bring you good tidings of great joy, which shall be to all people.*

*11 For unto you is born this day in the city of David a Saviour, which is Christ the Lord.*

*12 And this shall be a sign unto you; Ye shall find the babe wrapped in swaddling clothes, lying in a manger.*

*13 And suddenly there was with the angel a multitude of the heavenly host praising God, and saying,*

*14 Glory to God in the highest, and on earth peace, good will toward men.*[4]

For Mary, the scripture in Luke is a story of manifest hope and love for all people. She loves the season of Christmas. Whether it be finding the right pine tree, setting it up in our home, or putting an angel at its peak, the preparation recalls her mother's desire to always remember the true meaning of Christmas. If asked, she can tell you with vivid memory the origin of each carefully placed ornament. In keeping with her mom's traditions, Mary enjoys giving gifts that she has made, which include homemade jams and jellies that she makes during the summer months. An occasional well-made pie is another favorite.

Decoration would not be complete without placing an electric train to encircle the base of the tree as she had done so many times in childhood. It is a treasure to be with Mary at Christmas.

She shared with me the love of classical music. She endeared herself to my father with her quick recognition of Schubert's 5th Symphony playing on the stereo in the background when she was visiting.

The chocolate cream pie she had made for dessert also increased his appreciation of her qualities. Traveling up Route 8 along the Farmington River to hear the Boston Symphony at Tanglewood in the Berkshires, brought us close as we experienced the joy and beauty in classical music. One of the fondest memories of our early relationship was lying on the lawn there, listening to a live performance of *Appalachian Spring* by Aaron Copland. Mary and I were happy and relatively care-free.

As we stared up at the sky, Mary described her view of the rabbit on the moon:

"Listen, Wendel, it's a rabbit, not the man in the moon. The feet are at seven o'clock and the ears are at two o'clock. It is like one of those standing bunnies we used to get in our Easter baskets. I don't know how people see a man in the moon!"

Mary is one of those rare individuals whose imagination allows her to see such things vividly.

"Mary, I can see the spots, but a rabbit?" I responded.

"It's a beautiful night, the stars are bright, the moon is full. Can't you see it?" she asked.

It was never as clear to me as it was to her.

Mary's imagination and creativity have always been much more developed than my own. She loves *The Velveteen Rabbit*, written by Margery Williams in 1922; it's a story of a little boy's treasured stuffed doll that comes to life because the boy really and truly loved him.

"*The Velveteen Rabbit* is very real to me," she would tell me. It is a story of how love brings transformation.

Mary attributes her strength of character to her mother's unshakable love for her. Her father disclosed his sentiment that of all his children, Mary was best able to take care of herself. She is extremely capable and has always been loving, kind, and patient with me. She believes that charity begins at home and that it is important to know when you have enough. She is loyal to friends and faithful to family.

After graduate school, not able to find a position in my field of study, I entered the workforce as a professional painter. I went to work for Mary's father, who owned a paint contracting business. In the time I painted with him, I was a support to him in his business. He gave me the opportunity to learn a trade as I waited for the eventual job opening at the Environmental Protection Agency. He and I had a wonderful relationship. As I continued to pursue leads toward employment in the sciences, the painting business offered a modest income and an opportunity to learn the skill.

During the two years I painted, the hours were long and hard, but rewarding. The physical demands were extreme. Factory work with more than one water tank to paint was the norm and included sandblasting and swing stage operations. Residential and church work offered different challenges that required a refined execution and precision. The whitewashing of a roller coaster or the occasional painting of a firehouse gave some variety to the work.

One of my more interesting experiences I had painting in Mary's father's company was a job of replacing the finials in the bell tower of the First Church of Christ, Congregational in Farmington, Connecticut. My family and I routinely attended the church there after moving to Farmington in 1966. Mary's father's company got the job because the church knew of his company. Mary's brother used a boson's chair to replace the wooden finials with white plastic ones. I helped him by lowering the finials to the ground from the bell platform in the tower. After two years of intense physical labor, I was able to hoist a 40-foot ladder with ease.

I also became interested in butterflies. I had always been fascinated by them and spent much of the remainder of my free time watching them, catching them, collecting them, and mounting them in displays in my home.

Mary and I would spend lazy afternoons during my time off listening to classical music with her family. Mary played the flute. Ted played the trumpet with the Springfield Symphony in Massachusetts; John, the youngest of the six brothers, played the trombone; Bob played the French horn; Vern played the trombone;

and Greg played the trumpet. Ted, Vern, and Bob all played in the Army Band. Mary's memory of Ted's playing Haydn's Trumpet Concerto and our hearing it in times since has always transported us back to a simpler time. I learned of Mozart's Flute and Harp Concerto while at home with her and fell in love with it.

On my 25th birthday, just before I was to receive my Master's Degree from the University of Illinois, Emily shared the following Langston Hughes poem, "Dreams," to wish me well in my hopeful search for a job and my exciting future with Mary:

*Hold fast to dreams*
*For if dreams die*
*Life is a broken-winged bird*
*That can not fly.*

*Hold fast to dreams*
*For when dreams go*
*Life is a barren field*
*Frozen with snow.*[5]

— Langston Hughes

When not working, my time was taken up with filling out job applications, one of which was for a position at the Environmental Protection Agency.

Chapter 6

# First Year at The Environmental Protection Agency

IN 1977, I BEGAN working at the Environmental Protection Agency in Washington, D.C. The post was perfect for me: working to protect the environment. My formal higher education had begun on the hilltop of Cornell College in Mount Vernon, Iowa. There, my initial interest in English literature that had begun under the mentorship of a high school humanities teacher soon gave way to an interest in the sciences, especially the subjects of embryology and organic chemistry.

I liked the methods used to study the sciences, and the rigor of scientific investigation. At first, I was attracted to the premedical program and its curriculum of genetics, physics, and organic chemistry; however, the birth of Earth Day in 1970 marked a change in the focus of my activities from the study of medicine to the study of the environment.

I graduated from Cornell College, receiving a Bachelor of Arts degree with a major in Biology. I subsequently pursued graduate studies in zoology and environmental engineering, receiving a Master of Science degree at the University of Illinois. There, I became interested in the study of limnology, freshwater biota, and model aquatic ecosystems, and their application to the real-world study of how chemical pesticides behave in aquatic environments and bottom sediments.

When I was not in school, I would go to a local stream bed and look for aquatic invertebrates under the rocks in the stream. This was my enjoyment, and I did it routinely for about year. I was accustomed to going to the same stretch of river because of its proximity to my home. To my surprise, one summer afternoon, the stream had been channelized with concrete embankments. The stream was adjacent to a corn field and my understanding was that the channelization was necessary to improve field runoff from rainstorms. There went my tiny ecosystem. It was so easily done.

Channelization of a small stream may help in controlling runoff from plowed agriculture fields, but it destroys the natural beauty, the species makeup, and the ecosystem of the stream. I was naive to think that the tiny ecosystem could be saved, but I was horrified to think of how easily larger ecosystems face the same doom.

I was well-trained and well-suited for my task at the Environmental Protection Agency; however, the experience there was profoundly different from the two years of painting in Connecticut. The adjustment was a challenge: small town to big city, familiar to unfamiliar, small family business to big impersonal government, physical activity to cerebral endeavor, outside active labor to inside cerebral effort. It was difficult going to work and, yet, once beginning, I couldn't stop the work I struggled initially to engage: learning the program of pesticide disposal.

The structure of the office was not clear to me and the events were fast-paced. The amount of paper frightened me. The disconnectedness within the office isolated me from colleagues and new acquaintances. Initially, I had difficulty with the required drafting, typing, editing, and the mass of paperwork.

Regulations and regulation writing were new to me. I was involved in writing rules for and in disseminating information about proper pesticide storage and disposal. The constant deadlines were oppressive. I found it difficult to take a break from my work, even when my mind needed to refresh in a moment of silence.

I was uncomfortable being alone without a task to perform, working through expected breaks in the workday and bringing work home at night. When I did take a break, I would frequently leave the EPA building without any place to go. I felt alone, boxed in by a disabling condition of which I was not yet aware.

The building seemed a maze in which I had no space for myself. As I learned my job, I never felt I knew enough to be successful, which led to frustration and anxiety. It seemed I had no voice in solving the problems at the office or in the environment. I felt pushed and pulled by perceived pressures. My feelings of trapped panic over imposed deadlines, rushed turmoil over personal organizational issues, and constant exhaustion in trying to complete tasks, left me drained, harried, confused, and defeated.

Working at home after long days at the office became commonplace, the result of being overwhelmed at the office and feeling the need to escape to "buy time" to finish the work. Even though home was a familiar and friendly place, I was no more able to work there, because the problems had to do with my state of mind, not where I was. When I was alone and feeling hurried, I would work to exhaustion.

As I went to bed and tried to sleep, I would lie awake for long periods of time, obsessed with the coming pressures of the next day.

Daybreak would find me wrestling with another round of the same pressures as I got up to face the new day. The first thing I would do was reach for a cigarette. I was not aware of the reality of what was to come.

In an early experience that I had at EPA working on the pesticide disposal program in the Office of Solid Waste, I was responsible for the collection of all information, literature, official reports, and meeting notes for the Kepone pesticide spill in Virginia's James River at Hopewell. The collection was substantial; when the information was stacked sheet by sheet, it towered just above my shoulders.

The assignment lasted about a year and then I was assigned to be responsible for the collection of one-page pesticide damage cases reported from around the United States. After collecting the reports over a number of months, this collection, when stacked sheet by sheet, stretched to nearly the ceiling of the room. I was left to make a fundamental decision about the kind of work I wanted to do: did I want to be an expert in the study of one aspect of EPA's concerns, or did I want to be exposed to many problems? I chose to enter their contract program, which afforded me an opportunity to explore many issues. I stayed with EPA contracting for 38 years.

I worked with users, manufacturers, state programs, and regulators of pesticides, usually in the Midwest. This sometimes required business travel to the sites of activity, something that was also new to me. I was involved in determining the causes, the extent, and the remedies for pesticide contamination of the environment. Requests for assistance about alternatives for safe pesticide storage and disposal came from the government, the public, and private organizations. These new activities and responsibilities weighed heavily on me. Even Mary was unaware that I was struggling with the burden.

In addition, the long days and commuting by bus and subway were becoming overwhelming.

On an early spring day in 1978, I rested during the lunch period under a small tree down on the waterfront in Southwest D.C. near Fort McNair, the U.S. Army facility that is located between the Potomac and Anacostia rivers. I sat quietly and ate my lunch alone while watching passers-by enjoy the setting. I found myself reflecting on Psalm 23, a comforting experience, but strangely out of place in my anxious existence.

## Mary

*In June 1978, Wendel had been working for the U.S. Environmental Protection Agency in Washington, D.C. for about one year. He seemed excited about his position and had few complaints. The commute by car, bus, and Metro (subway), resulted in very long days and seemed more taxing than his job. I was working at George Washington University and also found our long days exhausting at times, but we were young and very excited to be working in and living near the nation's capital. Wendel's parents seemed proud of his achievement, something which was very important to Wendel.*

## The Power of Prayer

On one occasion at home, I was upset. Coming up the stairs from the basement, the Lord's Prayer entered into my thinking. Arriving at the top of the stairs where Mary stood, I found that my anger had been transformed and the upset gone. Afterward, I was mystified by the effect that the prayer had had on my attitude at the time.

In the weeks immediately preceding my psychotic break, I was working feverishly to finish an article I was asked to write for a national magazine about the use and eventual storage and disposal of pesticides associated with the maintenance of golf courses. It was an honor to be asked, but I felt inadequate to the task. As the deadline for submission approached, I became incredibly anxious. The article was eventually published, but at the time, I was being swept into the darkness of schizophrenia. I was smoking heavily.

Section 3

# Journey Out of Loneliness

### The Loneliness

*In the beginning, a stark realization of life;*
*not knowing where to turn.*
*Eye and ear gave no answer.*
*The interior realm not yet searched;*
*discovery and divine disclosures*
*yet to be made.*

*Existence seemed to be exactly that,*
*no sense of the Holy.*
*Forgotten was the love I had*
*known as a child.*
*Silent noise resounded within.*

— Wendel L. Miser
February 23, 2001

Chapter 7
# The Loneliness

## The Medicine

The medicine made me gag. When I got out of the hospital several weeks later, I came to the realization that my life had irrevocably changed. The medicine to keep me functioning in the world I had known was difficult to swallow, physically and emotionally.

**My body, my mind, and my emotions were locked in a battle against the schizophrenia that attacked my hold on reality and against the very treatment that was keeping me functioning.**

I yearned for a vaguely-remembered normalcy that existed before my illness and the medication for it began; but I could no longer remember what I was like before.

The side effects were challenging. My mouth was constantly dry, requiring me to drink fluids excessively to relieve a drug-induced thirst, a simple and ever-present reminder that I was no longer the person I had been just a few weeks before. When I would forget to take one of the medications to counteract the side effects of the main drug required to control the psychosis, my neck and face would tighten, unable to relax. At times, I felt that I was going to crawl out of my skin.

## Mary and Dr. Maloney

It was a daily struggle, a battle with an unseen foe within me that I could not have won without the love and support of my wife, Mary. Her commitment to battle the illness with me was unwavering and remarkable. In spite of this love and support from my wife, I felt profoundly alone, isolated in a condition that disturbed my reality. Mary experienced the loss of her normal husband, friend, and lover; she, too, was isolated by my condition and the demands of my treatment.

### *Mary*

*Things seemed better after Wendel was home and back to work. He was struggling and trying to cope with normal life, helping with chores around the house. Shortly thereafter when my parents were visiting, Wendel went out to mow the lawn. I was inside preparing lunch. Fifteen minutes later, Wendel came in, complaining that he could not get the lawnmower started.*

*Frustrated, I stomped out of the house, exclaiming to Wendel, "I can't do everything!"*

*I grabbed the starter cord. With one angry yank, the lawn mower started. We looked at each other in horror, Wendel because the mower started, and I because it started. If only it had not roared to life! I felt that I had made Wendel feel useless, just when he was trying so hard to regain his place in our lives together and in our marriage.*

*One day I was married to a budding Environmental Protection Agency professional and the next day I had a schizophrenic spouse plopped in my lap.*

*I realized that Wendel was really very ill. We worked*

*together on his recovery every day, especially on his medications. With the help of his psychiatrist, we were able to get his medications regulated, but it was difficult. We did everything together. We got frustrated together, angry together, disappointed together, and happy together.*

## Loss

I had lost the sense that there was anything fun to do with Mary: a swim, a tennis game, a bicycle ride, an ice cream cone. We made a few attempts at getting physical exercise together that included quiet walks in the evening. They proved to be futile.

Mary was left with the stark realization that my care was "all up to her." Most often during my early treatment, Mary questioned it. Her time was suddenly consumed with protecting my health: taking me to doctor visits, going to the pharmacy for new medicines, and constantly reminding me to take them. When I was not working, I was sleeping at home to avoid what I needed to do. Mary's frustration with me and my condition was palpable. It was a long time before Mary fully trusted and came to believe that I was in good hands with Dr. Maloney.

I couldn't feel comfortable in the present. Inwardly, I would mourn my broken past and my inability to remain in the present. Doubt consumed me. I was extremely awkward in social situations, often feeling trapped by those circumstances and wanting to flee from them. I was engaged with neither activities nor people at this time in my life; I was reacting to them. Maintaining normalcy was difficult. I wasn't doing chores around the house. I would mow the lawn only on a sporadic basis; however, it was always hard for me to start the machine. Mary would have to help me, affecting my sense of my own manliness.

In the months following my mental break, intimacy with Mary was very difficult. The idea of having children was a retreating thought for both of us. Only later in my life did I realize, that at a time when I was the most sexually able, I was the most distracted by my constantly challenging mental state. This led to anxiety, frustration, and compromised feelings for both of us about attempts at pregnancy.

### Mary

*I felt that we were often quite alone in the struggle. There were times that we had to persevere without a psychiatrist, without our families, without a friend, and for me, even without God. (I recognize now that He was always there, but I did not have that assurance then.)*

*The medical terms were all new to us: psychotropic, carbonic anhydrase inhibitors, Stelazine, Cogentin, Thorazine, tardive dyskinesia. Wendel and I were just trying to figure out the doses of medicine, the side effects, the adverse reactions, the unfamiliar feelings, the emotions, and the unexpected results. At times it seemed to us that the doctor and nurses looked at us as if we were drugged. In fact, Dr. Maloney was always there for us.*

Chapter 8

# The Struggle to Stay Well

EARLY AFTER COMING TO the Agency and shortly after my break, I met a new colleague, Jim, who saw my struggle and befriended me. He and I would take extended walks at the lunch break, discussing the newness of the Agency experience for both of us. He empathized with me and encouraged me to "let go" of the work in the evenings and to pace myself during the day. His companionship was comforting to me as I shared my feelings of anxiety with him. He quickly became a strong support to me in my daily routine as I coped with my job.

My illness was very difficult for my parents, especially my mother. She struggled, just as I did, trying to understand its origin in my life. She felt guilty for the horrible condition that had overcome me, and she attempted to cast blame to relieve the uncertainty of the origins of the condition. This guilt and blaming by my mother resulted in Mary's isolation just when she needed support and love the most.

Over the next five years, several recurrences of overt symptoms often seemed just below the surface of my daily routine. Early in that period, I twice ended up back in the hospital when the daily, ever-present medicine failed to produce the desired effect, a reminder of the serious and potential threat to the normalcy for which I longed. I visited my psychiatrist, Dr. John Maloney, once or twice every week, again a reminder of my vulnerability. But he also represented my path to recovery. The ups and downs of my illness sometimes resulted in many unscheduled visits to Dr. Maloney to adjust my medications.

There were many times when the medicine, its side effects, and the illness itself made me feel unlike I remembered feeling at any time prior to my breakdown. This led to outright combat between the medicine and me. With Dr. Maloney's guidance and Mary's insistence, the importance of taking the medication prevailed. I often did not want to take the medication, but I took it.

As I became frustrated with the medicine and my physician for prescribing it for me, Mary's frustration with me would grow. She knew how essential it was for me to comply with the medical regimen if I were to achieve any semblance of normalcy, even sanity. The difficulty was that I didn't know how I was supposed to feel on or off the medication. My sense of what was normal had been lost.

In spite of this, Dr. Maloney artfully adjusted the medicine and counseled me what to expect, gradually increasing my ability to take responsibility for my own medication administration. As the dosage stabilized and the therapy progressed, I came to terms with my need to take the medicine reliably. I began to appreciate the benefits of the medication for me and for Mary, even when the side effects stood in the way. It took a long time.

Chapter 9
# The Family's Response

## Mary's Father

My disease affected Mary's father in a profound way. At the time of my break, he was terribly hurt by what happened to me. Attempting to reassure me he said, "You are not crazy; you are just confused." He never turned away from me and was always kind, reassuring me that I was doing better every time he visited. He spoke of having great hope for me and my life.

### *Mary*

*My father was very supportive of Wendel. Although he had limited education and no medical training, he had what Wendel needed most. He showed Wendel compassion, especially early in his struggle with schizophrenia. He and my mother, who was slipping into early Alzheimer's Disease, provided support to me the best they could.*

## Uncle Wendel and Our First Home

By 1980, Mary and I were in the market to buy our first home and my mother's brother, Wendel, came to Virginia to help us do so. On the day of the closing, I was excited, but extraordinarily confused.

After the closing, plans were made to return to our apartment for lunch. We were in two cars and I was driving one of them alone.

I had misunderstood our plans and had no idea about what had been decided. I found myself quickly lost and disoriented as Mary and Uncle Wendel went on ahead in the other vehicle. This was in the age before cell phones, and I had no immediate way of contacting them. After driving aimlessly for a while in an attempt to calm down and get my bearings, I did recognize a street corner I knew in relation to the apartment and made it back safely. At the time, I had no idea of the agreed-upon plan and that I had been lost for more than 45 minutes. Mary and Uncle Wendel were relieved when I appeared at the front door.

## Andy

After my break, this new reality of my illness and its treatment brought feelings of separation between my twin brother and me. Andy and I were no longer connected. Although we knew this separation was real, we never discussed it. The feelings of individual loneliness for each of us were profound. Initially, we did not know how to reconnect to each other and to the happiness of the relationship we remembered. We hurt. And our remembered collective identity as twins dwindled. Andy was painfully absent from my life.

Our relationship was in uncharted territory. Before the break, we had primarily experienced ourselves as twins and our individual identities had been obscured in that relationship. My illness, however, brought an end to our simple childhood concept of our twinness. We were forced out of our sense of being twins, and into a recognition that the two of us were separate individuals. Andy was healthy and I was not.

I not only experienced the loss of my health, but also the loss of my twin-ness with Andy. We began to realize the impact of our separateness, just as the locked door of the Quiet Room of my first hospitalization initially had demonstrated the reality of the distance between us. I had longed for Andy's OK from the other side of the glass.

Responding to the illness, we found ourselves for the first time very different from each other. We were scared: for ourselves; for each other; for our life together as twins. I was not able to deal directly with these new feelings. Andy tried to find balance in his life, to be normal. Even before my illness, he had begun to celebrate his differences from me. But he ached seeing me suffer.

Because we are identical twins, the possibility of the illness happening to him was also quite unsettling for him. Fear pushed him away from me; he did not want to have the condition affect him. On the other hand, having the disease and the confinement of its relentless confusion, I yearned to be more like him. I perceived him to be free and stable.

Actually, Andy was neither happy nor at ease, because he saw me as possibly never again experiencing happiness. He feared he would never experience his normal twin again. This caused him great sadness. As he recognized his own need to become a fully functioning individual, he suffered, knowing that I might never achieve that for myself. He desperately wanted it for both of us. I had little happiness and the road to find it was obscure. We were both unhappy.

### Andy

*It occurred to me that, sometime around when Wendel went into the hospital, I had made a life altering and quite unconscious decision that I would never be completely happy. It went something like, "If Wendel is never going to be happy, then how can I be happy?" I saw that I had actually decided back in 1978 that Wendel would never be happy. Not after what had happened. So, in my world at that time, I had "sentenced" both of us to unhappiness. I would never again be happy, and neither would he.*

*I realized that the actual facts of what had happened in 1978 were far less significant than the profound meaning I had attributed to those events, a meaning which had caused so much suffering for me over the years. From the fundamental decision that I would "never" be happy, I had developed a way of being that was rooted in resignation and hopelessness, which I covered over with a thinly disguised pretense of being OK.*

*I could hear myself say:*

*"I'm happy... not really."*

*Or, "I'm fine, not really."*

*And then there was the unanswerable question that was always lurking: "Am I OK?"*

*Outwardly, I got along, I made do, I was successful, and I was making it. Inwardly, I was hopeless and angry. This was not the way life should have gone. I was helpless and not really happy. I pretended that everything would be OK. I hoped it would, but I could never be sure. In my heart, I knew it was not.*

*I often hid the fact that I was really terrified, vulnerable and hurt, not to mention completely hopeless. Once I saw I had been pretending that everything was "OK" and "fine"* for years, I started to be aware of the impact this had had on my life and on others for the better part of 23 years!!

The first impact that I became aware of was just how angry I was. Man, I was pissed off. After all, what happened never should have happened. I saw how the "should" and "shouldn'ts" of my life robbed me of my happiness. When I was being, "I'm happy, but not really," there was no way that I could experience real happiness. It was unavailable, out of reach.

In addition to being angry, I had been despairing, sad, and frustrated, particularly with Wendel. Then, I'd be hopeful that things would get better. I would be helpful, I would listen to him, I would be patient and loving, but there was always something missing, incomplete. I came to realize that I would make Wendel wrong for being the way he was. I made him wrong for letting this happen in his life. I made him wrong for not getting his life together. I made everything wrong. I made myself wrong for being the way I was being with him.

I wondered whether what happened to Wendel could happen to me. Months after these events, I would experience anxiety, sometimes in the middle of the night, waking up abruptly and suddenly in a state of anxiety. When this happened, Martha was always there, calmly and lovingly letting me know that things were "OK." But, I was never really sure.

As the years went on, Wendel saw his psychiatrist regularly. He made steady and good progress. During those years, I was studying as a psychologist at the University of

Connecticut. I saw powerfully that, for years in Hartford, I was reluctant to come out and let people know I was a twin. I often did not let people know that Wendel even existed. When I did, people would invariably say:

"Really, I didn't know that."

Then they would ask, "Are you identical?"

And even though we are, I would always equivocate by saying, "The doctor never established that with certainty. Our placentas were fused together and they never did any chromosomal analysis."

This was bull. The truth was that I could not say to people, "I have an identical twin. I am just like him!"

I was hiding Wendel from others. I was ashamed of what had happened to Wendel. I was concerned about what people would think of me. It was all about me. I'd get angry that I even had to deal with this. Why did I have to deal with this?

I had hardly ever shared my life with Wendel. I had grown up inside of the "twin thing" that I was not sure I wanted any more. I certainly did not acknowledge our "twin-ness" very frequently. Being an individual was more important. The sad part was that these years were the years in my life of having children and building a career, generative and satisfying to a degree, yet Wendel was not often included. I often felt separate from him. Actually, what I realized was that was the way I had wanted it.

For 23 years, my life was about being different from him. "I am Andy, not Wendel. Wendel is not Andy." I wanted to be known for whom I was, for my accomplishments, for my achievements. I knew as twins growing up, we were always *being compared. I wanted to avoid that. In many ways, I had shut Wendel out.*

## Work

It continued to be a struggle to work as the job continued to be overwhelming and demanding. I found it difficult to set priorities for my work and to complete projects in a timely fashion. I was required to coordinate large projects under tight deadlines that strained my ability to organize the work. On the medication, it was difficult for me to concentrate, making it even harder to complete my tasks at hand.

My illness also affected those around me at work. They didn't know how to engage me as I struggled, their fear and uncertainty sometimes as real as my own. I ate alone. I smoked alone. I walked the streets of Washington alone, but with a constant companion, the psychosis that haunted my hold on reality. I had no sense of peace, no sense of the Holy, no direction, and no purpose. I had no sense of hope. In despair, I tried to find my way alone.

Over time, however, as the medication and the treatment began to take hold, I became more effective, and my experience at work became less forbidding.

## Emptiness and Separation

Although I had grown up in a Christian home and had regularly attended church with my family, my break with reality and the demands of its treatment to keep me sane, initially abrogated the possibility of finding spiritual truth for my life. I felt that if my whole being did not pay attention to itself, I would be drowned in a sea of uncertainty, leaving me unable to function in a world that was streaming around me. I was overcome by work and the need to cope with the details of my daily life. God was not on the radar screen; I had forgotten about the God I had learned about as a child. I heard about religion on TV, but it was not real to me.

As I emerged from the initial few months of my illness, I began to sense that there was a void in my life, a deep chasm of emptiness that held no meaning, a separation from a God I once knew. My spiritual nature was enveloped by the darkness of my illness and obscured by my constant struggle to maintain a hold on reality. The separation I felt was profound: separation from the life I had known, from my twin brother, from my wife, from my colleagues, from my God. Televangelism was not saving me spiritually or medically.

I yearned for the familiar, which I had lost after the onset of my illness. One place I found it was in the books I remembered my father had had in his house and office during my childhood. I had been aware of many of the classics, just by their proximity, even though I had only read a few. After my break, I would buy many of these classics, not on the thought that I would read them, but because of the assurance that they would bring me to a place of familiarity.

## Music

Andy always encouraged me to see the possibilities of life and gave me assurance that there was hope to be found in this world. I loved Andy and yearned to be part of his life. He, too, felt the loss of his normal brother. Andy introduced me to the music of John Denver, and I found comfort in his lyrics about loss, struggle, and finding grace.

Music had been an important part of my life as I grew up. Now I needed soothing for my turbulent existence. The music of John Denver seemed to bring meaning where I had none and companionship to my loneliness. But I continued to sense a void in my life. I was still haunted by the separation and loneliness I felt, in spite of Mary's love and care, my psychiatrist's regular attention and commitment to me, and my family's love and support.

I listened for hours to the songs for words that would bring meaning to an experience I could not understand. Although the music was soothing, I could not find the assurance for which I longed. As I coped with this reality, one thought constantly came to mind: that of singing someday. John Denver's singing offered an example to me and the possibility of my expressing myself in a new way.

# Chapter 10
# The Conversion

*24 For I will take you from among the heathen, and gather you out of all countries, and will bring you into your own land.*

*25 Then will I sprinkle clean water upon you, and ye shall be clean: from all your filthiness, and from all your idols, will I cleanse you.*

*26 A new heart also will I give you, and a new spirit will I put within you: and I will take away the stony heart out of your flesh, and I will give you an heart of flesh.*

*27 And I will put my spirit within you, and cause you to walk in my statutes, and ye shall keep my judgments, and do them.*

*28 And ye shall dwell in the land that I gave to your fathers; and ye shall be my people, and I will be your God.[6]*

Ezekiel 36:24-28
King James Version

*38 For I am persuaded, that neither death, nor life, nor angels, nor principalities, nor powers, nor things present, nor things to come,*

*39 Nor height, nor depth, nor any other creature, shall be able to separate us from the love of God, which is in Christ Jesus our Lord.*[7]

Romans 8:38-39
King James Version

## The Preparation

It is my brother Jim who started me on my road to a relationship with Jesus. Jim and his family came to Washington to live after Jim accepted a position at the National Institutes of Health. During the four years that Jim was in the area, I didn't see him a great deal, but there was a time when we were together that was to be life-changing for me.

One weekend in the Spring of 1983, Jim asked me to join him at his home to help him paint his dining room. I had begun to watch TV evangelists and other programs about Jesus and had become inquisitive about Him. As we prepared the room for painting, Jim took the opportunity to tell me of his experience and love for Jesus. Reading from the Bible, he shared some well-known passages, most importantly for me, Romans 8:38 and 39. As he finished reading, I was moved to ask him the truth of the passages. He said with certainty that the passages were true and I have taken him at his word ever since that day.

These verses from the Bible became for me an assurance that, initially, I only vaguely understood. But these words gradually brought a reassurance to my clouded existence that I had a purpose, that there was a God of love, and that I could not be separated from Him. In the subsequent days, these words began a lifelong yearning in me to find out about Jesus.

I dwelled on Romans 8:39: "Nothing can separate me from the love of God."

This was becoming increasingly reassuring for reasons I didn't yet know. Who was this God? What was this love that could touch me and reach into my life of loneliness and despair?

## The Commitment

One year later.

"Come with me down the hall to the room on the right," beckoned my friend.

Dave knew that if I would catch just a glimpse of God, that I would be His forever. He knew that I was suffering, he knew my loneliness and despair. He knew the emptiness of my life. Dave had been patiently waiting for an opportunity to share his Lord with me. We went down the hall to a private room and prayed together. There in that small room, he told me about Jesus and how Jesus was the only solution to the questions and problems in his life. He told me of his own personal relationship to this Jesus. And then he said to me:

"I am going to pray for you to accept Jesus as your Lord and Savior."

And he did. For so many years, I had needed a new direction. In the past, many had pointed the way, but I had doubted until this prayer was simply given by my friend.

"Go outside and find a quiet spot on the grounds of our building," he said. "Sit and be with God. Be still and ask the Lord into your life."

I wanted to honor his request, but I hesitated. What was going to happen if I did such a thing? I was confronted with an immediate, awkward uncertainty: "Do I really want to do this?"

After mustering a certain level of courage, we parted and I went out. But I was frozen in time with his request. Looking around, I remembered a church nearby with a bench outside that was just across the parking lot. On its cornerstone were engraved these words: "I am the Chief Cornerstone." I walked there and sat on the familiar bench, a place that I had made a home in the loneliness of the years before. I rested and waited, but knew that there was a conscious, prayerful decision to make.

"When do I do it?" I pondered. "Now?"

The loneliness was still there.

"No. I'll wait."

Yet I knew that I was going to do it. Gradually, my mind quieted. I was still and a peace came upon me. I closed my eyes and said the prayer in the name of Jesus, asking Him to come into my life because I needed Him so desperately. When I opened my eyes, the world appeared the same. I felt the same. I was the same, or so I thought. I returned to the office, wondering what had happened, if anything. I couldn't discern any change. There was no lightning bolt, at least not for the moment. Days passed and nothing seemed different. Yet, I had asked the Lord into my life.

My friend would occasionally see me and offer encouragement.

"Come with me to Bible study," he requested.

Again, I was hesitant. But one day I found myself following along. I had been asked many times before and had sometimes gone. But this day was different: there was no hesitation. Once there with a group of eight welcoming new friends, I read the Bible aloud and the words came alive to me in a way that words from common books had never done before. The words of Paul to the Romans and the words of Ezekiel gave me vital assurance that God was with me in my struggle.

Jim continued to nurture my spiritual growth. After my salvation experience, I continued to struggle, however. The schizophrenia was a continuing, constant battle and ever-present companion.

My spiritual journey was beginning.

### *Mary*

*As Wendel began his search for God in his life, I, on the other hand, was looking for God in all the wrong places. Sunday morning televangelists only sharpened my skepticism.*

# Journey to Joy

### Healing Embrace

*In the middle of life,*
*a shattering*
*can open it to the Almighty*
*initially searching for anything*
*that would bring meaning.*

*The Lord standing close all the while*
*waiting for a time renewed in weakness,*
*beckoning the son toward home.*

*"I am the door," He said to me.*
*"Come to me, you who are weary,"*
*He said to me.*
*Listening, I have discerned*
*in these days of healing*
*my realization of His presence with me,*
*giving me renewed strength and confidence.*

*A mending:*
*He and I.*
*His life to praise;*

*my life to live in peace.*
*Love is recognized in surrender*
*and the resurrection.*

— Wendel L. Miser
May 4, 2000

Chapter 11

# The Beginning of The Journey

*3 And he humbled thee, and suffered thee to hunger, and fed thee with manna, which thou knewest not, neither did thy fathers know; that he might make thee know that man doth not live by bread only, but by every word that proceedeth out of the mouth of the Lord doth man live.*[8]

Deuteronomy 8:3
King James Version

*27 Peace I leave with you, my peace I give unto you: not as the world giveth, give I unto you. Let not your heart be troubled, neither let it be afraid.*[9]

John 14:27
King James Version

### I Have Not Known How

*I have wanted to live.*
*I have not known how.*
*I have been afraid no one will understand.*

*I have wanted to love.*
*I have not known how.*

*I have wanted to listen.*
*I have not known how.*

*I have wanted to understand.*
*I have not known how.*

*I have wanted to forgive.*
*I have not known how.*

*I have wanted to be patient and compassionate.*
*I have not known how.*

*I have wanted to give and help much.*
*I have not known how.*

*I have wanted to be real and authentic.*
*I have not known how.*

*I have wanted to sing.*
*I have not known how.*

*Teach me Lord.*

*This I do know:*
*I have been in prison and you came to me.*

*To love you and praise you makes all things possible.*
*I have wanted to live.*
*I now know you have understood.*
*I know you will teach me how.*

*Amen.*

—Wendel L.Miser
October 15, 1998

## Reverend Underhill

Shortly thereafter, Reverend Wayne Underhill, a Methodist minister and father of a high school friend, came to visit me. The medicine was beginning to clear my mind enough for me to work. He came to share with me about his love of Jesus and to offer comfort to me. At the end of his visit, he handed me a small card depicting God's right hand holding a child with His fingers over the child's left ear. On the card was inscribed Isaiah 49:16:

> *16 Behold, I have graven thee upon the palms of my hands.*[10]

For the first time, the oppression of the deafness in my left ear began to diminish. I also began to understand that God would bring healing to my life. I have carried this card with me ever since.

## Nick

We met Nick shortly after moving to Washington, D.C. in 1977. He was finishing his residency in ophthalmology at George

Washington University, where Mary had begun working as an ophthalmic technician. When he opened a practice, Mary was hired by Nick to manage his practice and to be an ophthalmic technician.

Most importantly, Nick shared my journey with me. He closely watched over the medications I was taking. He was always there for me and for Mary to comfort and advise. He supported us, enjoyed us, spent time with us, cooked with us, relaxed with us, but always was concerned about my medical condition. He spent hours with us relaxing after performing surgery, counseling us along our way. He has been a supportive older brother to Mary during the loneliness of her journey with me; he has been a confidant to me. He cares about people and he cares about us.

## *Mary*

> *Nick, my employer, an ophthalmologist with a brilliant and wonderful sense of humor, often helped me get through the agony of my situation, losing a healthy husband and gaining an ill individual who was very dependent on my support.*

## My Friend

For me, Nick embodied the excellence of a dedicated physician and the compassion of a friend. During my journey, we took many trips together: to Corinth where I stood on the platform where Paul had taught the Corinthians centuries before, to the Vatican where the beauty of the Christian church is gloriously portrayed, to Athens where we were embraced by his family, and to the Greek islands.

## Mexico

My mouth was constantly dry, a side effect of the medicine. In 1979, as Mary started working at the George Washington University in the eye clinic, we had invited a trainee at the clinic who was from Mexico City to live with us for a short time until she could find a place to live in the area. During her stay with us, she invited us to her home in Mexico.

I was on Stelazine and Cogentin at the time, very early in my treatment. The flight to Mexico City was uneventful. When we arrived in the city, I quickly realized the difficulty of finding suitable water to drink. I suffered, trying to keep my lips and mouth moist and my thirst quenched. Early one morning, there was a knock at our door and there in the doorway stood our friend with two glasses of fresh-squeezed orange juice.

"This cup of orange juice is incredible!" I exclaimed.

## Eva

One Christmas in the early eighties, it was bitterly cold. We were slated to go to Connecticut to visit family shortly after the holiday. The evening before we were to leave, I had gotten myself overly concerned about how much had to be done to be ready for the early morning flight the next day. The Christmas tree had to be taken down and the ornaments put away. Mary and I had to pack and the cat had to be quarantined.

As the evening progressed, a sense of panic set in. Still smoking, I was preoccupied with the possibility of causing a fire. With a live Christmas tree in the house, I imagined accidentally setting it ablaze and felt that we needed to get it out of the house as soon as possible. Although Mary tried to reassure me that this was not going to happen, I continued to perseverate. In the middle of the evening, I started to unplug everything: the lights on the tree, the toaster in the kitchen, and various lamps, thereby making it dark in most of the rooms of the house.

At the time, we had an indoor cat. In my confusion, I left the back door ajar, and much to Mary's horror, the cat got out. I was in my underwear when I impulsively went next door to our neighbor, Eva, whom I summoned for help to get the cat back inside. The Christmas tree was still up; the rooms of the house were dark; the cat was outdoors.

With Eva's help, Mary did get the cat back inside. Mary then calmed me down, although by the end of the evening, she was exhausted. We made the flight the next day, but I was frazzled.

## Mary's Mother

In the mid 1980s, Mary's parents began a tradition of coming to Virginia to live with us several times a year. This continued until shortly before Mary's father died in June of 1992. During this time, Mary was caring for her mother, whose health was failing due to Alzheimer's Disease. I was beginning to do reasonably well and was able to help out with matters around the house. Although it was hard for Mary to see her mother this way, I believe it was good for her to have her parents in our home.

On one occasion, on an autumn day at home in Connecticut, early in her mother's battle with Alzheimer's, we watched as she spent an afternoon quietly typing President Abraham Lincoln's Gettysburg Address by heart on her manual typewriter. Mary's mother loved me and over her lifetime, she imparted to me her sense of patriotism by proudly reciting the Gettysburg Address from memory many times. In doing so, she told of our honored dead and a nation's resolve for renewed freedom. She spoke of her love for her country and her unbroken faith demonstrating her authenticity, and her grace. She would sing *Silent Night* in German and the hymn, *Nearer My God to Thee,* one of her favorites.

## Journaling: The Beginning

Gradually, ever so slowly, I began to have a sense of God's peace in my life. My fractured experience was helped by structure. Andy shared with me the importance of being organized. I have used an organizer for many years, a structure that has provided security and reassurance to my journey. At the time, my mother provided strong spiritual support and guidance for me. Even though I sometimes found myself in conflict with her, I never doubted her love for me, especially as I emerged from the darkness of my schizophrenia and as I began my life-changing spiritual journey.

In 1983, I began to journal. The journaling not only became a chronicle of my recovery, but was also therapeutic in my spiritual journey and important in my healing.

Jesus had just entered my life in a real way and I had a deep understanding that I had found what I was looking for. This realization served as a catalyst for my journaling about Christian concepts. It proved to make all the difference.

## Carlos

A few years later, I met Carlos, who had the same professional position that I had—Contracts Project Officer. We worked closely together on contractual matters, helping the office develop a vibrant program centered around the use of outside contractors in support of the office's environmental programs. I shared with him my interest in butterflies and journaling. He supported me, promoted my journaling, and listened to me reading it to him. He also encouraged me to share my butterfly interest with him.

"Study them, read about them, increase your knowledge," he would say. "Become an expert!"

He would also encourage me to read from my journal on a daily basis to become grounded in devotional concepts.

His interest was gardening.

"Be like a reed; a reed does not question the wind that bends it," he said to me, reflecting his relationship with God.

"When we retire, we will plant rutabagas together."

Our time together was often spent in a bookstore, reading books. Very often I would leave the store with a new inspirational book from which to learn. Carlos was interested in me and shared my journey.

When my father died, he counseled me by saying: "Time softens all the edges; heals all the wounds; dulls all memories."

## The Train Ride

I was traveling alone on a train from Washington, D.C. to New England to meet Mary who was already in Connecticut. On the train, I sat down next to a young man who engaged me in conversation,

"Where are you headed?" he asked.

"I am visiting family in Connecticut and meeting my wife in Hartford," I responded.

"I am off to a music camp for gifted individuals, situated in northern New England, for a month of piano lessons. I am really looking forward to the next month," he said, genuinely excited about the opportunity.

"Who is your favorite composer?" I asked.

"Chopin. I especially enjoy playing his waltzes," he responded.

I was becoming comfortable with him and our conversation. We talked for quite a while and then fell silent. Then, in the middle of our conversation, feeling safe with me, he announced:

"I am a schizophrenic."

I was paralyzed. "So am I," I wanted to respond.

Immediately, I realized that I was apprehensive being with him and from that point until I disembarked at Hartford several hours later, I remained that way. Why was I uncomfortable being with him? Why couldn't I share with him that we had a common experience?

Chapter 12

# The Journey Continues — 1

## My Struggle with The Diagnosis of Schizophrenia

Dr. Maloney initially described my condition to me as severe anxiety. Our discussion of the term schizophrenia came up much later in my therapy. I think Dr. Maloney always wanted me to discover the truth for myself. The connotations of the word itself and the societal implications for the individuals who have schizophrenia were difficult for me to accept. It was years before I accepted myself and the condition I constantly faced.

I said to Dr. Maloney, "I may not outlive this condition."

To which he replied, "Oh, but you may outlive worrying about it."

## Nolean

In 1986, I met Nolean at the Waterside Mall below the offices for EPA Headquarters. She is an incredibly hard working, energetic individual who makes it clear to her colleagues, "I am not doing this work for you, I am doing this for the Lord."

Shortly after I met Nolean, I was walking down the hall at EPA, still with my head down, my troubled spirit slumped, confronting my schizophrenic condition.

"Hold your head up, Wendel," she said, "Jesus loves you and SO DO I."

At that time in my life, I was not sure whether anyone other than Mary loved me, or whether I even loved myself. Now I knew Nolean loved me.

An African American, she grew up in Central North Carolina, one of 14 children born to a share crop farmer. When Nolean was young, her mother would ask Nolean to put her shoes under her bed each night before she went to sleep. She did this so that Nolean would kneel in the morning to get them. Her mother would say to her: "As long as you are on your knees, pray to God for blessing."

Nolean exclaimed: "Wendel, my family didn't have much money and we lived off the land, but we were rich in spirit. All we had was hope in Jesus. I didn't have time to be lazy growing up!"

"I am sure that you have never been lazy in your life," I responded.

Her father wanted Nolean and each of her siblings to be a success, but most importantly, he wanted them to put Christ first. Nolean told me about her involvement in the Civil Rights Movement. The story of the Greensboro Four is well documented in American civil rights history, chronicling four African American students from North Carolina Agricultural and Technical State University who were refused food service at a Woolworth's lunch counter in February 1960.

In September 1963, Nolean started to attend the university. That Fall, she went into the store, sat at the same lunch counter, and witnessed the same prejudice against African American customers. In the years before President Lyndon Johnson signed the Civil

Rights Bill into law in 1964, there was much unrest on and around the campus. Nolean found herself in the middle of the storm.

I met Dr. King in 1963 at the age of 12 and began a deeper understanding of the Civil Rights Movement and its importance in the United States.

As I struggled, she assured me, "You are forgiven; Jesus purchased your forgiveness on the cross; your life has been saved."

And, "There is still room for you at the cross."

## Smoking

After 18 years, smoking had gotten the best of me. I couldn't concentrate; I couldn't work effectively. I was constantly exchanging my feeling of anxiety and tiredness with the experience of smoking another cigarette, which led again to more anxiety. In 1986, I paid $225.00 and entered a program to quit smoking sanctioned by the American Cancer Society. The program was a series of positive reinforcement exercises and positive self-image reflections that sustained me. I stopped smoking. The six-week program has paid large dividends in improved health and a greater sense of my physical self ever since. I was beginning to feel better.

## Church

I continued in my Bible study, coming to a deeper understanding of my relationship with God and my personal relationship with Christ. The individuals in the group brought insight to the scripture, and the regular study of God's word gave me constant reassurance of His love. After a number of years, I gradually began to sense the need to be in a Christian community of friends in order to grow in my walk with God.

In 1990, I began to attend the Rock Spring Church in Arlington, Virginia. The associate minister there, coincidentally, had just moved from the Congregational Church of Farmington, Connecticut where I had previously attended with my family. Encouraged by my mother to attend there, Rock Spring is where my Christian life and service began to mature. I served on the deacons, oversaw the physical plant of the church, and grew as a worshipping Christian. Mary, curious about the church, followed me there in 1992. In one of his sermons, the minister spoke words that were very meaningful to me as I struggled on my journey:

"In our deepest despair lies the seed of our strongest faith."

My faith was growing.

## Classical Music

In 1990, I also began to listen to classical music again. Partial deafness is a condition with which I was born. Early in school, I was aware of neither my deficit nor the distinctions other children with good hearing were making. When my hearing loss was discovered, I chose not to pay attention to it. I did not consider myself to be hearing impaired; however, I was only passively hearing the music and missed much of its beauty.

Later, I joined the choir at Rock Spring and began to sing sacred and classical music, a developing passion that I shared with my father. Dad had sung in a number of choirs and listened attentively to opera, classical music, and religious works, often following their scores. By sharing this love of singing with him, we drew closer together. Because of my illness, it was especially important for me to have his approval, even more than when I was a child. After listening to one of my performances, his acknowledgement of the excellence of my music meant a great deal to me. My continued journey toward health now included these experiences of classical music and singing.

## Thomas

I met Thomas Small in 1993. Thomas was a security guard for the newly occupied Environmental Protection Agency building. Although he didn't carry a gun and was not physically imposing as he patrolled the lobby of the EPA, he had a deep spiritual presence.

An African American, Thomas was a minister in the Pentecostal church. Thomas always had time to spend with me, if only a few moments. His perceptiveness allowed him to look into my life, see my anxiety and doubt, and minister to me. We would often spend lunch together, a spiritual break in the middle of the work-day. Thomas magnetically drew me to a secure place where I could easily share my struggles with him. Encouraging me as I was going through my tribulations, he told me:

"Jesus loves broken vessels because he loves the joy of restoring them, filling them with his Holy Spirit."

As I searched to understand the importance of God in my life, Thomas said to me:

"Man creates religions; God wants relationships."

He also said: "The Lord has dominion over this world. You are with Him, and with Him and through Him, you are protected. The world has no dominion over you."

Thomas' words gave me great comfort as I faced my fears and anxieties each day. As I tried to cope with my anxiety, he claimed for me:

"He (the Lord) is more than able, be anxious for nothing."

He also said: "Bring your mountains to me (the Lord) and I will melt them like wax."

One day, seeing me walking down the hallway, obviously feeling better, coming out of one of my funks, Thomas exclaimed, "That is the Wendel I know!"

I also asked for some advice: "Thomas, I have been journaling for 12 years. What shall I do with it?"

"Call that Chapter One and start Chapter Two," he responded.

Several days later, Mary's mother died; that afternoon, I began Chapter Two. My earlier journal had been more a reflection of my listening to friends in Bible study and writing down important truths about Jesus. I would reflect on scripture by writing down favorite passages as my understanding of the Bible began to grow. As I had traveled around Washington, I would notice church signs and bumper stickers exhibiting Christian themes and record them in my journal.

As I started Chapter Two, I began to take my journaling as a serious exercise of healing and quiet reflection. I began to pay particular attention to what was happening to me as I learned the teachings of Jesus through the Bible and through the church's sacraments and songs. I catalogued the growth in my understanding of the message of Jesus and my response to it by establishing chapters with titles reflecting my response.

Throughout, I learned of the promises, the teachings, and the miracles of Jesus. Shortly before my father died in 1999, I came to a profound sense that I had been healed. From that point forward, my journaling reflected my attempt to express the faith and joy I now felt through my relationship with Jesus.

Thomas' influence on me was similar to the impact of my brother Jim. As I confronted my feelings of worthlessness, Jim reassured me:

"You are worth the death of His (God's) Son."

I often felt shame and embarrassment that I had suffered a nervous breakdown, which had resulted initially in behavior I could not control. As I slowly but surely recovered, my journey was a commitment to make progress one day at a time. Jim encouraged me:

"It is not that you fall down, it is how you get up."

## Allen and Kirby

I met Allen and Kirby in the middle of my career. In very different ways, they were both interested in leadership and motivational techniques. They both helped me to "get outside myself" and to broaden my outlook and relationships with people. Allen was also one who journaled Christian concepts. Our common experience deepened our friendship. Allen said to me:

"The magnificence I see in you reminds me of the Lord's hold on you."

I told him that I felt the same about him. When the Lord imparts magnificence, you can feel it and see it in others. This conversation went on between the two of us for quite a while and when I would see my friend, I would see his magnificence and he would see mine. We would laugh full of joy at our realization held by grace. I was not surprised, for I knew that it was the Lord's doing for both of us. Divine love sparked magnificence deep within us, lifting our companionship ever higher.

Kirby counseled me on time management, workload management, and my working relationships in the office. Kirby helped me quit smoking. He taught the American Cancer Society course on smoking cessation that I had attended.

## Bob

In 1995, Bob, one of Mary's older brothers, came to live with us as he pursued his dream to become a full-time actor. Acting opportunities in New York were dwindling and he was attracted to some options in the Washington area. During his stay with us, he and I became very close; he was a great support to me. Bob sang in some of his professional dramatic roles and he was the first person to encourage me in my singing. His initial instruction helped me to graduate from passively listening to music to actively participating in music by singing. The first major piece of music I sang after joining the Rock Spring choir was Schubert's Mass in G Major. The beauty and complexity of the music and its score were intimidating.

"Sing out, Wendel, don't worry about what you sound like," Bob admonished as he stood by me, listened to my voice and sang with me, steadying my efforts as I gained confidence.

His voice was quieter, but stronger than mine. I was just beginning to open a door to God through music and singing.

Bob was also an avid baseball fan and had gotten me interested in the Atlanta Braves. His love for the Braves began when the franchise was in Boston as the Boston Braves. He continued to follow the team when it moved to Milwaukee and subsequently, to Atlanta. Holding his scrapbook, Bob recounted:

"I wept when the Boston Braves lost the World Series in 1948 to the Cleveland Indians."

Eighteen months after his arrival in our home, Bob, his son, Geoffrey, and I traveled to Atlanta to attend a Braves baseball game.

On the way home, he developed tingling in his left arm. A subsequent MRI demonstrated a malignant brain tumor for which he underwent treatment with surgery, radiation, and chemotherapy. Although the therapy arrested the growth of the tumor temporarily and he improved briefly with physical therapy, his remission was short-lived.

Bob's son, Geoffrey, 14 years old at the time, spent time with his father in our home shortly before Bob died. In May 1998, Geoffrey wrote this piece in tribute to Mary's caring for Bob:

## Sacrifice

*Moonlight glistened off the blanket that covered my*
*sleeping Father as I entered his room one night.*
*The light reflected off the guardrails of his bed and*
*my still-sleeping eyes squinted for a second.*
*When I stared back at the room,*
*I noticed my Aunt Mary huddled in a white blanket*
*On the floor to the side of my father's bed.*
*She slept there like a sentry guarding my father.*
*I thought of my Uncle Wendel, upstairs in bed alone,*
*A witness to the sacrifices my aunt had made*
*for a family that would not forgive her.*
*My father rustled in bed and my aunt awoke for a second.*
*She looked over at the bed, but did not notice me*
*Standing in the doorway.*
*She rested again, as my father fell back to sleep.*
*I turned away and started to walk back to the couch*
*Which had been my bed for the last few weeks.*
*I looked back for a second and took in the image of*

*A person who could help someone without a word…*
*And dreamed of a family that would be willing to respect that.*

Caregiving for Bob was challenging for Mary, especially confronting Bob's extended family.

Shortly before Bob died, he entered hospice care. He died peacefully on a bright and glorious day. It was a beautiful day to go to heaven. I gave Bob's photograph of two of the most famous Braves pitchers, "Spahn and Sain and pray for rain," to Geoffrey.

### Emily

*I heard from my mother often, but her way of expressing about Wendel's condition never helped me to become any clearer about his illness. At some point, I knew that Jim was helping Mary and Wendel and that gave me the peace of mind to know that someone knew what to do.*

### Andy

Andy had started his career as a licensed psychologist working with patients who were mentally challenged. In the middle of his career, he worked as a marriage counselor. Subsequently, he began coaching individuals to see possibilities for their lives. He has a talent very different from my own. His personal growth included participating in life development and leadership courses. As early as I can recall after my break, even as he inwardly dealt with his feelings, Andy would speak to me of the possibilities in my life. It took me a long time to relate to what he was offering me.

*Andy*

*Although I did not like what I was seeing, there was a truth being revealed and I was starting to feel free. What I saw was that others, including Wendel, his wife, Mary, my family members, as well as my parents-in-law could never be sure that I would be real with them about what was going on in my life. They could not trust me to be fully honest, open, or truthful. I had shut a large piece of myself away from me and from them. My guard was up. After all, I was pretending to be happy, pretending to be OK, and nobody was going to find out what was really going on. I saw clearly that I had successfully shut everyone out. I was not letting anyone in. I was alone. I often heard the little voice in my head say, "I will never be happy."*

*Much later, I saw something quite extraordinary. I realized that I was the one who had made the decision that I would never be happy. The events of 1978 and those that came afterward did not cause me to be unhappy. I had already made a decision I would never be happy and I had already decided Wendel would never be happy either. I had done this, not Wendel! It had been something I had decided. It had been all mine.*

*The circumstances did not cause this. Rather, I had made a fateful decision about my life. I had sentenced myself to being unhappy with no real possibility of satisfaction or fulfillment. I had made Wendel responsible for my happiness, not me. I had done that. I was stunned at first when I saw this, and then overwhelmed. I burst into tears, uncontrollably sobbing, letting go of all the years of holding, retreating, hiding, faking, and pretending. There was a moment I thought I would not stop. I did not want to stop. The tears were cleansing. They were warm and forgiving, loving, and embracing. As my sobbing completed, I was enveloped by love. An image of Wendel was there, kind, gentle, and forgiving. I was back home. Just Wendel and I were there, whole, complete, and loving. I was free and so was he. We were one again.*

*I called Wendel, who was in Washington, D.C., and he answered the phone. Not knowing where to start, I said to him:*

*"Hi Wendel, I have something I would like to share with you."*

*I told him what I had decided for my life back in 1978 and how that decision had left me feeling about his life and how that decision affected my life. On the phone, I declared to him my responsibility for that decision and I told him that he was "off the hook."*

*I asked him if he would forgive me for the way I had been with him over the years. I had no certainty in that moment how he would respond; however, Wendel let me know that he really knew how I had been all those years and that he had forgiven me "a long time ago."*

*In those precious moments, I was aware of his grace and his forgiveness. Wendel for me occurred as a giant, a magnificent and magnanimous human being. He had forgiven me. He had forgiven my ugliness, my deceitfulness, my separateness, my pettiness, and my smallness. In his forgiveness, I was returned to myself and to my humanity. He had accepted, in an instant, something in me that I had not done for him in 23 years!!*

*I told Wendel that I loved him and that I was proud to be his twin brother. I let him know that I had spent years trying to be different from him. I declared to him that I was like him. I embraced our twin-ness. In that moment, not only was I home, but he was home with me. It was an unforgettable transformational moment.*

*In the weeks that followed, I shared this with his wife, my mother, my sister and her husband, my parents-in-law, and my wife. What opened up in my life was a realness, an honesty, a truthfulness, and a happiness that filled me with the experience of fulfillment and joy. I really was happy. The future was wide open. For the first time in years, I experienced being satisfied and fulfilled in my life. All kinds of new possibilities for living were opening up for me.*

## Coin Collecting

In the 1970s, Andy and I expanded our collection of U.S. and foreign coins and he bought metal containers to house the major coins of importance. Andy was the keeper of the collection in the 1970s and 1980s when he added many foreign coins.

After my break, Andy knew that I needed to get interested and involved in something other than my immediate concern for office work. I began to reconnect with him. He decided to give the coin collection to me to work on. He determined that it was a way for me to become focused on something that had been very important to both of us earlier in our lives.

As a result, I became the keeper of the collection in the late 1980s as Andy encouraged me to become interested in it again. I have added to it a little. We have an almost complete set of Mercury head dimes, all except the dime that would make the collection worth much more—a 1916 coin minted in Denver. We haven't gotten it yet.

## Trip to Hawaii in 1998

Zyprexa was approved by the Food and Drug Administration in 1996 for treatment of psychiatric disorders. I began the transition from Stelazine to Zyprexa about 18 months later as we were planning a trip to Hawaii. Mary knew that there might be trouble. As we prepared for the trip where Mary was to attend an ophthalmology meeting, my anxiety increased, and my paranoia exacerbated.

I had been on Stelazine and Cogentin for almost 20 years. I had coped with the neck muscle spasms by balancing the Cogentin against this side effect of Stelazine and the dry mouth, a side effect of Cogentin, by drinking copious amounts of diet Coca-Cola. The transition to Zyprexa was proceeding gradually, but the effective dose for me had not yet been achieved as we took off to the airport to fly to Honolulu. Mary was acutely aware that the transition from Stelazine to Zyprexa was not yet complete.

On the way to the airport, the husband of the couple who took us to the airport, a male nurse, noticed my distress and said to Mary:

"Are you sure you are OK to go?"

"I think once he gets to Hawaii in a relaxed environment," Mary responded hopefully, "he will be OK and have a good time."

But on the plane, placed next to the window by Mary in order to be somewhat isolated from the other passengers, I announced to her, "I need to turn myself in to the authorities."

I contemplated using the airplane telephone in the seat console to notify the FBI. I continued a constant stream of paranoid concerns about what I thought I had done. Mary's hope that my arrival in Hawaii would result in a reduction in my anxiety didn't materialize. Once in the hotel, I was anxious about going out. I stayed in the room while Mary attempted to attend her professional meetings, but then I felt confined. On the third day, I confronted Mary:

"I have to get out of here!"

The Zyprexa wasn't fully working yet.

Realizing my distress, Mary tried to advance our return to Washington, D.C., but was unable to change the reservation. Frantically, Mary spoke with Dr. Maloney, Jim and Nick multiple times on the telephone. In consultation with my psychiatrist in Washington, the dose of Zyprexa was increased and I got through the rest of the week. To shorten the time on the airplane, we decided to break up the trip by stopping for several days in California where Jim and his family were living at the time.

"I will be there to meet you in the morning," Jim had reassured me. His words were the only thing that allowed me to get on a plane the next day to the West Coast where he was waiting for us.

On arriving in Los Angeles, I was better, but still anxious, still subdued and still experiencing paranoid ideation. While with Jim and his family, Stephen, one of his sons, nine years old at the time, noticed my distress and anxiety, and followed me out of the kitchen.

"It will be all right," he reassured me. "Wendel, I will pray for you."

This carried me through until I returned home and the full dose of Zyprexa had taken effect.

## A Choice to Make

After we got home from our trip to Hawaii, Dr. Maloney impressed upon me, "Wendel, you need to accept yourself, warts and all."

I knew that this meant I needed to accept myself as having schizophrenia.

Shortly thereafter, Dr. Maloney said to me:

"Wendel, you have a choice. You can stay in therapy because you are ill or you can stay in therapy to remain well."

I had a choice to make.

Chapter 13

# The Journey Continues — 2

**Trip to Naxos — 2002**

A day in Naxos with Nick was one of the happiest of our lives and left us enchanted for a lifetime. Arriving by hydrofoil around midday, we came upon the island amidst strong wind gusts off the water, which lasted all afternoon. A perfect day.

As we left the vessel, Nick went ahead to scout out a place where lunch could be leisurely enjoyed before the boat's departure to Athens later that evening. He found a table near the water's edge for an extended meal. The day was extraordinarily bright and cool; the warmth of the sun was balanced against the cold of the wind.

The open-air seating in the outdoor restaurant left us with a good choice of tables only yards from a rushing wall of water at the edge of the Aegean. It seemed that God's Spirit was moving about us. We had a chance to tour the various dishes and a wide choice of food; it was understood that the courses were to be brought to the table at long intervals of time. I could not help but think all was right with the world that day.

The wind continued to play havoc with everything, especially with the hat Mary was wearing, which she had purchased on the island of Santorini the day before.

"Mary, hold onto your hat," I reminded her.

As she returned from a short walk between courses, I recognized her hat as she came into view; my fears of finding myself alone all afternoon relieved. As we settled in, Nick summoned the waiter for hummus, tzatziki, dolmades, baba ghanouj, kalamata olives, and pita. Subsequent courses would consume the afternoon. Nick's presence with me, especially here in his own country, put me at ease.

For Mary, the day had an innocence that could not be harmed, a delight in simple grace. There was a cocoon of safety for her to feel like a child again: the cobblestones and bougainvillea, the ships in the harbor, and the fish. The day felt created just for the two of us, and Nick was our guide: white and blue, an island setting placed perfectly by the sea. The spray of white ocean foam rising against the shore gave its rhythmic impact, a momentary rainbow shown through the mist. The three of us were wholly alive as the equatorial sun marched across the sky, bathing the island in a light so bright as if to bring the reality of heaven closer to earth.

In late afternoon, Nick left us for a solo hike toward the "Portara," the island's gate erected in the sixth century, B.C., to honor Apollo.

"I will be back in an hour and meet you at the dock for the hydrofoil to Athens," he called to us.

Mary and I stayed at the table, reveling in the truly beautiful island visages until the hands of the clock got the best of us. In leaving real time behind, we had had a wonderful memory to savor. We made it to the dock only to wait for more than an hour for the hydrofoil to arrive. As usual, Nick seemed to know just when to return, as he arrived just as the ship was safely in port and accepting passengers. As we collected our things to board, an almost expected gust of wind came up, as others had that afternoon, and suddenly blew Mary's hat into the water, where it vanished into the surf.

## Mary

In the Fall of 2002, Mary developed colon cancer. Her cancer scared me. My life received a shock. The thought of living without Mary raised my level of anxiety, but I was reassured by Thomas.

"Wendel," he would say, "she will be there in the morning."

Mary had her own struggle, fighting the cancer. She had to undergo aggressive treatment that weakened her even as it cured her; however, to the present day, she has never wavered in her strength as a person. As she healed, I helped her and took her to the appointments with her oncologist where she received her chemotherapy.

I continue to learn from her. She is remarkable. She loves pistachio ice cream, the seventh and ninth symphonies of Beethoven, and the season of Christmas. She has always decorated the tree in our home by placing each ornament on each branch with such loving care and attitude. Most often, a model train has circled the base of the tree.

### Emily

*We would join them in Maine during those years and always had a wonderful time. Our children loved and still love their Aunt Mary and Uncle Wendel. They say that they are easy to be with and fun, though they called Wendel their "sleepy" uncle; he did sleep a lot.*

*Casual conversation was still not easy, but I connected with Mary and we enjoyed similar things. It felt right. I knew that Wendel had changed medications at some point,*

*and that some of them made him thirsty; he did drink can*
*after can of soda. And then in the early 2000s, there was*
*another medication that the doctor wanted Wendel to get on,*
*but it was proving to be a little difficult to switch.*

## Trip to Wales and Amsterdam — 2004

I was excited to be able to switch the medicine to control my symptoms of schizophrenia from Zyprexa to Abilify. Zyprexa had been a vast improvement over Stelazine and Cogentin, but the Zyprexa had stimulated my appetite so much that I had gained quite a bit of weight.

Dr. Maloney prescribed a gradual taper of the Zyprexa as I began to take the new drug, Abilify. Although transition to the Abilify was not yet complete, things seemed to be going well as Mary and I prepared for our trip to visit Jim and his family in Wales, and subsequently, Andy and his family in Amsterdam.

We were meeting Emily and her husband Jon in the UK before going on to The Netherlands. As we boarded the plane to cross the Atlantic, I was happy in anticipation of being with family and of the fun we were going to have, but Mary could see the warning signs of problems ahead.

On the plane, I again became acutely paranoid.

"Are you sure that you have the travel documents," I anxiously asked Mary, worried I would not be able to function.

Observing my increasing distress on the plane, on arrival in the UK, Mary alerted Jim that the schizophrenia symptoms were reappearing, precipitated by the change in medication and the long flight. Upon arriving in Wales, several hours after landing at

Heathrow Airport and unable to contact my psychiatrist, Jim re-instituted the therapeutic dose of Zyprexa in addition to the Abilify.

### Jim

*I was horrified and heartbroken. I had been looking forward to Wendel's visit and sharing time with him and Mary. My children also were looking forward to their visit with great anticipation. It was going to be a wonderful time with my brother and his wife.*

*Instead of experiencing a joyful visit, I realized that for the next week I was going to have to be his physician and psychiatrist rather than his brother, and Mary was going to be his nurse. Although I was confident, I was not sure we could get him back. I kept this to myself.*

*Several days later, I finally reached his psychiatrist, who agreed with the plan of care for Wendel. He, too, was confident that Wendel would recover, but cautioned that it would take a little time for him to emerge. As it turned out, it took the entire week. I realized that I was going to lose the time with him that I had been anticipating so much.*

## Suffering

The first two days in Wales, I was barely functional and very quiet. It was hard to be with the family and at one of the first dinners, I announced:

"I can't do this."

Then I got up and left the table.

Emily and Jon arrived two days later, but by that time, I had retreated within myself.

### *Emily*

*We took a trip to Wales and Amsterdam to be with Wendel and Mary, and Jim's family in the summer of 2004. When we arrived in Wales, we learned that Wendel's new medication wasn't working effectively yet and for the first time in years, we saw what his illness looked like.*

*He was shuffling around the house, usually following Mary, and unable to speak clearly. We couldn't really have a conversation and I felt afraid for my brother. Jim was confident that we could get him back on track over the few days we were there.*

*Experiencing Wendel's improvement was startling. As he began to talk again, he expressed anxiety about where his passport was or where Mary was. For the first time, I saw the anxiety that comes with his illness and felt a small glimmer of connection with him. I knew about anxiety with my own challenges. Maybe we were a little alike. Once the medication was really working, after a week, Wendel was back—more himself, communicating better.*

### Anxiety

After a couple of days, my orientation was better, but my anxiety was much worse. I needed to know where Mary was every second of the time. I stuck very close to her. On the third day, Mary went down to the kitchen without me. Realizing I was alone, I became acutely anxious and arrived in the kitchen wearing only my underwear. After finding Mary and realizing my predicament, I was then able to return to our room to dress. Later that day, we went to the local village with Jon and Emily.

As I sat with Jon on a village bench, I asked him, "Where is Mary?"

"Mary is in the store," he responded. "Do you want me to get her for you?"

"No," I answered, "I just need to know where she is."

I was getting better.

As I improved with the additional doses of medication, taken in consultation with Dr. Maloney in Washington, it became even more clear to Jim and Mary how close to psychosis I lived my life.

It was also clear that I was improving quickly. But I was very sad and felt very sorry for troubling Jim, Emily, Mary, and the family. I continued to feel sorry for the disruption I had caused, not fully aware of the love and concern of my wife, Mary, and my brother, Jim—the two who had orchestrated my care and recovery.

After a week in Wales, now recovering normalcy, Mary and I with Jon and Emily traveled on to Amsterdam to visit my twin brother Andy and his family. When we arrived, I had improved enough that Andy could not see any sequelae of the events of my psychotic crisis of the previous week. We had a wonderful time in The Netherlands, visiting the home of Anne Frank, taking trips to historic sites, and enjoying fun and fellowship with family.

The trip home to Washington, D.C. was uneventful. Jim and Mary, cognizant of the severity of my episode, were especially grateful for the rapid return of my normal state of being.

Section 5

# The Joy

*It has taken many years for me to have*
*an experience of God. To see and*
*experience my God. To realize that He loves me,*
*and by that love I can love others. That He wants me to*
*know Him and have a relationship with Him in a way*
*that I no longer imprison myself in my anxiety and*
*fear of what tomorrow may bring, but rather,*
*live in joyful anticipation of a future*
*embraced by Him.*

*I am amazed that I am here, but not surprised*
*why it took so long. I didn't know and*
*couldn't have known. Until now.*
*I now know that He is always faithful and*
*that His faithfulness encompasses every*
*realm of my life in Him. I now realize that I have an*
*essential relationship with Him that*
*cannot be broken by any power*
*known or unknown. I realize that to have a*
*relationship with Him will open relationships*

*with others — deeper relationships — the*
*extent to which cannot be foretold.*

*Faith, love and hope all have meaning now*
*that lend perspective for my life that I will*
*live in the knowledge that all is well.*
*But by thy grace go I with the absolute*
*knowledge that He cares for me absolutely*
*and that He is always and will forever be with me.*

— Wendel L. Miser
January 15, 1998

# Chapter 14
# The Experience of Joy

*Mary*

*I didn't want to do this.*

*The horror of Wendel's break was watching him suffer and the fear that he would one day slip into a psychotic episode from which he would never be able to escape, even with the help of doctors, medicine, and love.*

*It is difficult for me to revisit much of what Wendel has had to endure simply because he suffered a broken psyche. Had his arm or leg been mangled in an auto accident, he would have been surrounded with the compassion and goodwill of family and friends.*

*It is more than four decades since Wendel had his initial psychotic break. Since that time, he has had two episodes of far less severity, the most recent in 2004.*

*There are those, even some close to him, who regard him as "scary," a little "crazy." It hurts when someone is bothered by his tremor or occasional drool, both side effects from long-term use of medication. When it hurts the most, I remind myself that these are merely manifestations of a disease against which Wendel has so valiantly battled.*

## Music

Classical music is now an important part of my life. Dad had exposed me to the music of Dvorak, Saint Saens, Respighi, Beethoven, and Mozart. Mary shared with me the work of Haydn, Schubert, Copland and her favorites, Beethoven's *7th Symphony* and *4th Piano Concerto*. Schubert's *9th Symphony* was her father's favorite.

Music brings glorious colors to my days and to my experience with Mary. It also brings me great joy. While singing the great masterpieces, I have felt my spirit soar to the heavens. The intense beauty of the Requiems of Faure and Brahms, the *Christmas Oratorios* of Bach and Saint Saens open me to feel the magnificence of the Lord in song and the majesty of God. Rossini's *Petite Messe Solonnelle* and Schubert's *Mass in G Major* lay the foundation for me praising my Lord in song. Church hymns are equally important to me, whether sung at Christmas, Easter, or throughout the year.

The music of John Denver continues to move me to deep grace and peace, and to inspire me to sing to the Lord. I now realize that John Denver, through song, has been telling people of the wonderful possibilities of life.

He brought me to a shared sense of the environment, its creatures and its wonders, and helped me give my own voice to the protection of the environment. He raised my awareness of children and the impoverished worldwide. He gave me a sense of the real possibilities of life, just as Andy had done before I embraced Jesus. In the loveliness of his singing, John Denver passed on to me a beginning sense of profound personal peace and awareness of the Creator through his music, just as so many others had done in the telling of the gospel stories.

## Singing

In September 1998, I had my first real opportunity to sing outside my church choir in the New Dominion Chorale, a 250-member, mixed singing group that would routinely sing the great masterpieces of choral music. Deaf in my left ear, I never felt that I could "hear my voice"; however, on the day I rehearsed for the first time with New Dominion, the director asked his singers:

"Who wants to stand next to the new guy?"

One of them yelled, "I do, because he sings in pitch." On that day, I went from a fundamental feeling that I had to struggle to listen, to a feeling that I could improve my listening through singing with others. My self-esteem went through the roof.

Being with the group that first year began for me a life experience of stretching beyond what I had previously known. One of the most thrilling moments of my life came in June 1999 at the end of my first year with the group. At its annual meeting, the conductor announced his intention of forming a men's chorus and asked the men in the mixed chorus if any would like to join. I had always enjoyed men's voices and was thrilled to have the opportunity.

In March 1999, I had gone with my wife to the Kennedy Center to hear a local men's singing group, The Washington Men's Camerata, a group conducted at the time by the same conductor of the New Dominion Chorale. It intrigued me to see him conduct the Camerata at the Kennedy Center.

During the performance, I turned quietly to Mary and asked her:

"Why am I in the audience instead of being on the stage?"

In the back of my mind, I knew that I aspired to sing with such a men's group in the Kennedy Center. When the opportunity arose, I was thrilled. The National Men's Chorus was formed in the summer of 1999 and began rehearsals in the Fall. I was with the group during its 19-year existence.

## Baseball with Andy

I love baseball. So did Dad. Andy does also. I love to root for the underdog, an excellent trait as I currently live in the nation's capitol. Every year I have shared the agony of defeat of young, inexperienced but exciting teams with great potential: The Nationals.

Dad was a lifelong Red Sox fan, his life ending before they achieved the glory of their first World Series victory since 1918. Mary and I often now go to the Nationals' baseball games to enjoy the experience of the ballpark and the excitement of anticipating the potential success of a maturing ball club.

Andy always wanted me to go with him to the National Baseball Hall of Fame and Museum in Cooperstown, New York, to celebrate the rich history of baseball. In 1998, we watched an exhibition of the old way baseball was played with paddles and balls, and examined the memorabilia of the exploits of years past.

Just after visiting Babe Ruth's plaque in the "Hall of Plaques," we ate lunch at a corner pub. As we ate, a St. Louis Cardinal baseball game was playing on a small television. Our backs were to the television when the batter hit a home run. The pub erupted in jubilance and Andy and I realized in the same instant that Mark McGwire had just hit his 60th home run of the season, tying the Babe's home run record. We laughed together as we shared a passion for our national pastime.

## Andy

*Wendel and I smiled and laughed, and then smiled and laughed some more. It was special being in Cooperstown, experiencing the Baseball Hall of Fame, seeing Big Mac's home run and sharing this moment together.*

*We were there. We were the last two people who stood at Babe Ruth's Hall of Fame plaque before Big Mac tied his record. It makes such a great story. Wow! We talked about it for the rest of the day and all the way back to Hartford the next day.*

*That moment will connect me to Wendel forever, like so many other moments of our lives. That wonderfully magic moment connects me to what's important: family, brothers, and baseball. I will always remember where I was and with whom I was when Big Mac tied Babe Ruth's home run record.*

*I came to realize it was the relationship I now had with my twin brother, Wendel, that gave me so much happiness. I knew he was OK. I knew I was OK. I knew we were OK.*

*It is inside Wendel's grace and the love that we share now that I am a whole person, that I am satisfied and able to fulfill my dreams. It was in my completion with Wendel in 2001 that my life truly transformed. I gave up being different than he was and began to experience our likeness. Nothing really changed, yet everything changed.*

*I found out that I can simply embrace my life as it is, accept Wendel for exactly who he is, and come home to our relationship again and again.*

## The Dream

A month after our Cooperstown trip, I had an extraordinary dream about Andy and me, having a conversation with him. Here is the dream:

*It's early in the morning, Andy, and I have just awakened from a sound sleep. I've been dreaming about us... just the two of us, not constrained by anything imaginable, just the two of us playing with baseballs and a few bats.*

*The field is green and beautifully large. Very green trees line first and third. There is a tree behind short and a tree in right center. The trees seem appropriate for the space and they are green, leafy and large. The field is large, but close to us. The air is personalized by our companionship, you pitching and me batting. A number of balls fill a basket, white balls—boy, are they white.*

*You are close, pitching to me, understanding and wanting me to hit the ball. I swing, but the connection doesn't feel right... I'm going for the feel, not the distance. All the while, you are pitching lefty. I swing, sending the balls here and there, but the feel is not right. You are patient; you throw and I swing.*

*All the balls, now dispersed, you shag them... right, center, and left near the edge of the field, bringing them back in the basket, intent on me getting the feel right. You are with me... getting my feel of the bat... you pitch... I swing... the ball is lifted to right and my hands are soothed, assured, at peace.*

*The struggle has left me... only the grace of the moment remains. I am with you, Andy... the field is green; the balls are white. My hands are warm. You have stayed, always pitching, so I can get the feel right.*

## Journaling

Journaling brought further structure and clarity to my relationship with Jesus and the world. As I started my journal in 1983, only having a glimpse of Jesus, I felt profoundly broken. As I remained in therapy, I gradually realized the importance of keeping the appointments with Dr. Maloney and of continuing to journal.

Journaling has not only allowed me to stay focused, but also has allowed me to journey inside myself and in the Christian world in which I found myself. My journaling has provided me a place of peace and quietness. It is a place where I can explore and express my thoughts about my Lord and my God in an attitude of worship.

Christian writers have influenced my journaling. My favorites—John Stott, Oswald Chambers, and Max Lucado—have nourished me in grace. Journaling has significantly improved my writing skills and helped me to meditate on God's word. Journaling has also helped me become and stay well.

## Singing

In May 1999, just before my dad died in June, the New Dominion Chorale presented a joyful and varied program of American Music at the Vienna Presbyterian Church in Vienna, Virginia. As I stood in the chorus singing that day, the interior of the church seemed strangely familiar. In an instant, I recognized the space. I verified with my father that the church was my family's church where, at the age of nine, I had received my third-grade Bible. My family had lived in Vienna, Virginia from the early to late fifties when Dad worked as a civilian at the Pentagon.

My first concert with the New Dominion Chorale was Gioacchino Rossini's *Petite Messe Solennelle* with its glorious fugue *Cum Sancto Spiritu* performed at St. Luke's Catholic Church in McLean, Virginia. It was very exciting for me to be with the group.

After the concert, I was relieved and experienced extreme elation about the audience's acceptance of our performance. My time with the New Dominion Chorale has been an immersion into the choral music of the Great Masters—Bach, Handel, Mozart, Mendelsohn, and Brahms.

The National Men's Chorus was invited to sing with the Army Chorus during their 50th anniversary season in 2006. At its 10th year celebration in April 2009, the National Men's Chorus sang at the Kennedy Center with my family in the audience and me inwardly beaming on stage. What began as only a dream 10 years earlier, had become a reality.

Another joint concert with the Army Chorus in March 2013 celebrated the 150th Anniversary year of the Battle of Gettysburg during the Civil War. The fellowship of the group was wonderful. Being one among many over the 19 years was sheer joy. My experience of patriotism, my expression of the Holy, and my enjoyment of classical music have enriched my life. The National Men's Chorus took me places where I would not have gone myself.

Singing became an expression of my health and my joy, an expression of worship to my God, and an expression of my thanks to Him for bringing healing to my life. Singing requires me to be completely in the present, listening attentively to all the sounds that surround me. Listening in this way requires me to shut out the past and to avoid considering the future. Singing brings me peace, a peace that allows the careful listening required for the singing itself and a peace that silences the anxiety of my past. Singing also helps me overcome my deafness.

My inability to hear and listen has been superseded by a peace and stillness that has allowed me to hear the words of this world more clearly and to listen more effectively to this world and to my God. I can sing better and my pitch is better. This same discipline, learned in singing, has instructed my life: I can now live peacefully in the present without the oppression of past events or the fear of the future.

The experience and realization of still water has always amazed and comforted me deeply, whether I see it in a puddle, shallow pool, fountain, or lake. In recent years, after my discovery of our Lord, when I see still water, I always reflect that He has led me there. I remember realizing it for the first time.

I had, from childhood, been familiar with Psalm 23, but had had no personal relationship to it. In the hubbub of one Christmas season, I was getting ready to sing Handel's *Messiah* with my mixed chorus at the church where Mary's cousin and her family regularly attended near Washington, D.C. In the space just outside the sanctuary stood a fountain of strikingly beautiful still water. For a few moments, I was profoundly graced by it.

In the months after the concert, I would think of the words of Psalm 23 often and remember the years of noisy activity and anxiety that had left no room for the quietness of our Lord. Quietness came after years of therapy and after finding the grace of the Lord. Still water is a reminder that He is with me always.

## Dad

I needed to go to Connecticut to be with Dad. He was dying of colon cancer and I wanted to be with him. I had recently received an Office Excellence Award for my contract work in assisting with the success of EPA's Resource Conservation and Recovery Act National Program Meeting held at the Willard Hotel in Washington, D.C., and I wanted to share that with him. He was proud of my accomplishments; this was important to me. I also wanted to hear his thoughts after listening to the recent performance by my choral group of Brahms' *Requiem*, his favorite requiem. He recounted:

*Now this is a piece that goes way back for me. The first time I ever heard it was at Fisk University in Nashville, Tennessee, about 1936. The Black choir there was superb— and they had a director who had been trained in Germany. Soon thereafter, I acquired the score and used to play it over on the piano.*

*In Chicago in the early forties, I heard a white choir do it, but nowhere near as well as the Black choir at Fisk. When we were in Chapel Hill, we heard another performance in the Duke University chapel. Recently, I heard it here in Hartford at the Bushnell, but that is too big a space for the music to really get to you.*

*I particularly recall a time in the early forties when we spent a Christmas in Ashland, Ohio, where Uncle Harold's church had a particularly fine organist/choirmaster. At a Christmas Eve sing-along at her house, I brought along the score of the Brahms Requiem, which surprisingly, the lady had not seen before. With great enthusiasm, she tucked into it and we sang it all the way through at sight. A memorable evening.*

*Your mother and I found time last evening to sit down and listen together to the recording of your Brahms' German Requiem. It is a very fine performance of the work, and we enjoyed it very much. Your mother was moved by it. Your conductor clearly had a mature grasp of the music and its subtleties, and conducted a very professional performance. I liked the baritone soloist, but found the soprano, while very good, a bit below the ideal I have in my head from earlier times.*

*In case you think I am putting this on, let me say that I have had a Peters edition score of the work for over 65 years, and have played it over, and heard performances at various times and places over that time! The only thing about the performance that tended to put me off a bit from time to time was that, while I have the German words in my head for many passages, the chorus was singing in English. That was the right thing to do, of course, for an English-speaking audience, but for an old timer like me, not hearing the familiar words was a bit of surprise from time to time. You can tell your colleagues in the choir, and the director, that this old timer admired very much what was achieved.*

I wanted to share with him the love and joy that Jesus had brought into my life; and I did. The week before his death was a wonderful time together. In a circle of prayer around him with Mom and his minister, I prayed for him. And we entered into each other's experience in a deeper and more profound way than at any previous point in our lives.

My father said to me:

"Life is not a problem to be solved, it is a mystery to be lived."

I learned a lot from him. After one of our talks, he reaffirmed his belief in God and the Lordship of Jesus Christ. Shortly thereafter, he died. After his death, I realized that rather than this time being the beginning of my sadness, it was the beginning of my joy, knowing that my earthly father was at home with my heavenly Father.

In the planning for Dad's memorial service, I asked my mother if I could take Dad's place in his church choir on the day of its observance. It was an honor for me to sing in his choir that day, standing in his spot and harmonizing with the group as we sung together "How Lovely is Thy Dwelling Place" from Brahms' *Requiem*.

## Acceptance of My Diagnosis of Schizophrenia

I sought a better understanding of my condition, particularly after I saw the movie *A Beautiful Mind*, a true story about John Nash, a Professor of Mathematics at the Massachusetts Institute of Technology, a diagnosed schizophrenic, who eventually won the Nobel Prize for Economics.

As I saw his life unfold in the movie, I identified with his struggle with the disease. As the movie was ending, in the dark of the theater, Mary and I cried intensely. We both realized that my illness was a battle for both of us and was intensely real.

John Nash's story was a powerful one and enabled me to ask questions of Dr. Maloney about my relation to it. After seeing the movie, I felt free, freer than ever before.

## Work

When I retired, I had been with the Environmental Protection Agency for 39 years. For all that time, my efforts had been in pre-award and post-award contract activities. Program areas that I had supported included pesticide waste disposal initially, hazardous waste control and its regulation in the middle of my career, and municipal waste management in later years.

Recently, the office has embraced resource conservation and safe materials management as the Agency's waste programs have matured.

In 1991, on the day that Andy's son, Carl, was born, I received a Bronze medal for Commendable Service for work I had done with colleagues to improve the way contract management was executed in the office.

In 2003, I received an On-The-Spot Award from the Office of the Administrator.

In June 2005, I was given the Office's Contract Management Excellence Award for my contract activity, and in 2010, I received the Employee Excellence Award.

In 2013, I received the Customer Service Recognition Honor Award for exemplary customer service for my assistance to the staff.

In 2015, I also received the Operational Support Professional of the Year for the office. It was a rewarding career with many challenging assignments.

## Emily

My relationship with my sister Emily is new and exciting. Although she was a silent partner with me early in my illness, she has now supported me in my commitment to stay well, encouraging me to hold fast to my dreams.

## Emily

*During the past 10 years, I can say that I feel a much deeper connection with Mary and Wendel for a variety of reasons. For one, we are all older and wiser, and with that has come a yearning for connection. At least it has for me. We have all lost our parents and being together feels comforting and just right.*

*And, not insignificantly, Wendel has been on a medication that seems to be the best yet. He seems the most like himself (or the self that I remember from our childhood) in that he is communicative and engaging. I feel like this medication enables him to be much more present with all of us. When we are together, it is relaxed and easy. I had forgotten about Wendel's sense of humor and his love for his family.*

*I can also say that I have developed a deep sense of love and respect for Mary and her unwavering commitment to my brother throughout all these years of his illness. I cannot imagine what his life would have been like without her. She is a gift to us all. As we age together, who knows what life will bring our way in terms of our health and our lives. But I am certain now that we, as a family, will help one another and will not be afraid to ask the right questions when needed.*

*It has taken years for me to understand and be comfortable with Wendel's mental illness myself, but now I am less afraid and more at ease and committed to him. And for that I am grateful.*

## Andy

Now, many years later, Andy and I have returned to each other. We speak of our differences, but have returned to a sense of our oneness, not as childhood twins, but as loving brothers. We accept each other for whom we are, more so now than ever before.

Andy's health had been a context for my illness and loss of health. My road to wellness has allowed me to realize that Andy is now at my side and I at his. His promise to me at the time of my break—that I would someday be OK—has been fulfilled. His loss of a normal twin to illness has been transformed to the gain of a truly healthy brother. I am now OK. Today, my love for Andy and his love for me gives me the feeling of complete joy. This is also true for him.

## *Mary*

*Wendel says that I never made him feel that he was letting me down. Actually, he never let me down.*

## Mary

Mary and I have been married more than 49 years. Many of them have been difficult for her as she has had to be a caregiver, sufferer, and partner in my disease.

Although she has suffered great loss in the course of my illness, she has been essential to my recovery and healing from schizophrenia and has always insisted that we grow together. She is now truly my partner in life and joy, my lover, and my best friend. She is a fellow traveler on my journey and has remained fiercely loyal to me.

Although my illness offered Mary a unique opportunity to love and care, she could have retreated and left; however, Mary has persevered with me in the demands of my recovery. Frightened in the beginning, she remained loyal to me in our adversity. I discovered that when Mary becomes a friend, she becomes a loyal friend for a lifetime. Because of this, she has always had good friends to sustain her through her hard times.

Mary was always close to her mother, who would say to her: "Make the best of a bad situation."

> *"And suppose the world don't please you,*
> *nor the way some people do,*
> *do you think the whole creation*
> *will be altered just for you?"[11]*

— Phoebe Cary, 1882

Mary learned to persevere from her mother. She has always persevered, teaching me to do the same as I have overcome my disabling condition. Mary knew her mother loved her. Subsequently, Mary's love for others has been an expression of her mother's love for her.

"Love yields to circumstances, Wendel," Mary's mother would say to me.

Armed with this expression of love's perseverance in all circumstances, Mary's love has seen us through challenging times together. Her graciousness and kindness throughout my illness have been her most precious gifts to me. In my journey back to reality, it was Mary who most helped me to become human again.

With Mary by my side, I went from a mind of distorted thought to a stable single-mindedness by discovering faith in God in the life of the Spirit. The Holy Spirit has worked through Mary for the last 40 years.

## Nolean

Nolean, one of my closest friends at the Environmental Protection Agency, is a dynamic Baptist who exudes her faith in Christ. She is very outgoing and was always busy helping others in the office. Nolean takes care of people.

She made very clear to me, "Wendel, I've got your back."

I would try to see her each day, a magical person who lives out her love for Christ. She assured me that in spite of her own 40 years at EPA, "I'm not going to retire until you do."

She is a true friend. Recently, Nolean reassured me, "No matter what your circumstances, keep Christ in the center while keeping your eyes on Him, and He will show you which path to take. Just hold onto the hem of His garment."

## Thomas

As I came down to see Thomas at his front security station one day, he reminded me:

"He's got the timetable; he's got the clock; and Wendel, you are right on time."

These words gave me a wonderful sense of well-being that I was just where God wanted me to be all the time. Out of my illness, I have always felt very ordinary, nothing special.

Thomas claimed for me, "Jesus ordains ordinary people to become extraordinary people."

And our purpose is to serve Him. Thomas would also explain:

> *"Faith is the vault;*
> *Grace is the door;*
> *God's abiding love is the treasure."*

## Medicine: Now

### Mary

> *The care that Wendel has received from Dr. Maloney has had little to do with money and everything to do with a love for a fellow human being and a patient.*

## Health

I have been healthy now for many years; however, I still require medication and the twice-monthly supervision by Dr. Maloney to keep me well. With Dr. John Maloney's care, there is always a listening, an intense listening in the moment, a listening for context. It pervades the room where I sit with him; his manner and way of speaking are kind and steadfast.

My voice is heard and his interested response to me has been quietly consistent. Never impatient, or loud, he offers reassurance, engaging me to steady myself in the circumstance in which I find myself. His regimen is followed, my confusion is overcome and a path forward is found. My growth toward meaning, purpose, and faith is constantly being discovered and affirmed—nudging me toward the life I believe the Lord has wanted me to have as I learn to forgive and accept myself in a most profound sense.

I feel better now than I have at any time since 1978; however, the drugs have left me with a severe tremor in my left hand, a bother I endure. It is a small price to pay compared with the tremendous benefits of the medication: the relief of the symptoms of my condition and the sanity I now enjoy. On Abilify, I now feel completely normal.

With the decades of support from Dr. Maloney, I now feel more assured that I am in God's hands and that my life is a gift from Him (God).

I haven't smoked for more than 25 years.

## Transformation

Butterflies and their inherent beauty have always been special to me. Their growth from a caterpillar through the chrysalis to an adult butterfly in just 10 days is one of the true miracles of life. Their vibrant colors, from the brilliant yellows of the swallowtail to the golden oranges of the monarch, have always brought me great joy. Their transformation represents for me the possibility of my own transformation through the resurrection of Christ.

I am now complete in my God, having left my anxieties at the foot of the cross of Jesus. Although I temporarily lost my health and Andy experienced the loss of his normal twin, I believe with all my heart that there is no loss in God and that we can be triumphant in gaining His eternal presence. God has been faithful to me even as I have been faithful to Him. Out of my darkness, I have discovered the light of God.

I go to church most Sundays, sing in the choir, and support the church's activities with my resources, my energy, and my prayers. And I am absolutely sure that God loves me and that nothing can separate me from His love. I am sure that I am called to His purpose. I no longer worry about my life and my relationship to my God.

## Being an Elder

In 2006, we left Rock Spring for a new church experience at The First Christian Church, Falls Church (Disciples of Christ) in Falls Church, Virginia.

At Rock Spring, the service and communion were led by the ministerial staff. At First Christian, communion is lay-led by Elders. In the beginning of my experience at First Christian Church, my responsibilities included being a deacon. In 2014, I was invited to become an Elder. The experience of being an elder has deepened my faith. I feel I have grown in the experience, improving my leadership and public speaking abilities. It has blessed me immensely, especially preparing meaningful words for invitation and prayer at the Lord's Table.

On Thanksgiving Sunday in 2015, I offered these words:

> *Let our seeking rest on a foundation of prayerful surrender; and, our understanding rest on a foundation of knowledge and wisdom provided by the Holy Spirit. Let our individuality rest on a foundation of assurance that we are created by our Heavenly Father, and our community rest on a foundation of gracious and honorable acceptance of our differences. Let our trust rest on the foundation of God's Holy Word and our assurance rest on the foundation of God's promises. Let our faith rest on the foundation of God's abiding covenant.*

## Monoclonal Gammopathy

In October 2013, I was found to have a monoclonal elevation of a protein in my blood and was referred to a hematologist. Dr. Christie explained that at some point I might develop a hematologic malignancy or multiple myeloma. This did not change my outlook on life or what I did from day to day. I continued to work at the Environmental Protection Agency and serve as an elder at the church. I was checked regularly by Dr. Christie.

## Retirement

When I retired in January 2017, I received an American Flag that had flown above the Capitol, a letter of appreciation for my years of service from President Barack Obama, and a Service Citation from the United States Environmental Protection Agency. I will always cherish these gifts from my government, an acknowledgement that I had made a difference.

## Multiple Myeloma

In October 2017, I developed back pain and an elevation of calcium and creatinine consistent with the onset of multiple myeloma, a type of blood cancer. This was confirmed in January 2018 with a bone marrow examination that showed 20% malignant plasma cells.

When I was first told by my doctor about this diagnosis, I did not flinch. I had been told in 2013 that it was a future possibility for me. So, in a way, I had known it was coming since 2013. And now I was healthy enough to take it in stride.

I began the treatment for multiple myeloma in February 2018. There's a hard truth to it. Yet, I am safely in the hands of good doctors and my faith has not wavered. My family has been truly supportive. I am reminded of the biblical verse in Philippians 4:6-7 that reassures me of God's grace:

*6 Be careful for nothing; but in every thing by prayer and supplication with thanksgiving let your requests be made known unto God.*

*7 And the peace of God, which passeth all understanding, shall keep your hearts and minds through Christ Jesus.* [12]

The start of treatment, called an "induction period," lasted 17 weeks and consisted of three strong chemotherapy drugs, Lenalidomide, Bortezomid, and Dexamethasone: one a daily pill, one a once-a-week injection, and a third, pills given on the same day of the injection.

In addition, I was given an infusion once a month of a medication to reduce my calcium. For me, the induction period was relatively uneventful except for one small skin rash and occasional tiredness. I have been treated for more than four years and I am now in a maintenance period, taking a reduced dose of medicine in pill form.

I am not anxious. I do what the doctors ask of me and instead of worrying about the disease, I concentrate on the treatment regimen. I believe it's a very honest approach to a horrible disease and it allows me to be positive about my life as I cope with its reality. I go forward in peace and continue to be strengthened with Mary by my side.

Early on in Mary's own battle with cancer, she said something that resonated with me in the intervening years from then until now:

"You need to learn to live with cancer, not to die from it."

She is a little farther down the road, yet I am learning this with her help.

Early in Bible Study, the Lord told me in Matthew 17:20:

> *20 for verily I say unto you, If ye have faith as a grain of mustard seed, ye shall say unto this mountain, Remove hence to yonder place; and it shall remove: and nothing shall be impossible unto you.*[13]

Mustard seed faith sustains me and I believe my faith has made me well. I am now encouraged greatly after starting the maintenance period knowing my medical numbers continue to be normal. I feel that I have my life back and, again, I am thankful for what committed doctors can do with the treatment of difficult diseases.

Although potentially fatal, I have had a peace about the diagnosis and treatment that can only come from God and His love and protection. In the experience with two illnesses, I have been blessed by the love that has surrounded my recovery, by the healing power of medicine, and by my acceptance of Jesus.

It has been well worth all the hard work, continuous effort and perseverance. I have a better understanding of myself and a closer relationship with my family, friends, and Mary. Most importantly, I have grown closer to my Lord and God.

## Greater Appreciation of Life

When I first met Dr. Maloney, he told me that from his experience, schizophrenia was a young man's disease. At the time, there was profound hope in what he said. Throughout my struggle, I have developed discipline, commitment and perseverance, and an essential relationship with the Lord. My present experience is that all is well.

Recently, Dr. Maloney has been using the term "in remission" when describing my disease. Knowing this brings palpable excitement and joy to my life, as well as increased enjoyment in small things. He said to me,

"Aren't you glad to have met the challenge?"

I feel good and I am healthy. My calcium and creatinine are much improved. My physical challenges have not compromised my spiritual health. I continue to love the Lord and rely on Him for my strength. I am certain that my experience with schizophrenia prepared me for my next health battle. I am optimistic, but realize that I must commit myself to do the work necessary to control the multiple myeloma that has invaded my life.

For me, profound changes have taken place in my life. I am at peace; my place in the world is secure. I am more involved with the people around me and I have a deep appreciation of all I have been through. My marriage, my family, my work with the environment, and my singing bring me great joy. Today, I feel more fully human and I feel closer to my God than ever before.

# Afterword

## Love Waited

*Love waited for me to recognize it.*
*It then enveloped me as if my time*
*prior to my recognition of it never existed.*

— Wendel L. Miser
March 28, 2008

## Spiritual Healing

Once lost in the grip of disease, I am in relationship with Jesus and in the hand of God. Many years ago, with nowhere else to turn, I asked the Lord into my life after realizing that I needed him terribly. By doing so, that one prayerful knock at the door to eternal life changed my life forever. Years have passed since that time.

I know now that I have become an adopted son of my Heavenly Father and that I needed the saving grace of the Lord Jesus Christ. What followed was the realization that I was born again as His son through what Jesus had done for me on the cross.

This relationship with God through Christ makes me realize that I have always had a Heavenly Father who loves me unconditionally.

## Physical Healing

From my own experience, I know that schizophrenia is a treatable condition in the United States today. A major issue confronting sufferers of schizophrenia and the people who know them, is there often are no warning signs of a "first episode."

This was the case for me. My first schizophrenic episode was extreme: uncontrollable confusion, paranoia, anxiety, and fear. These manifestations in milder form can be seen as normal behavior, making the interpretation of the extreme symptoms of schizophrenia and the recognition of them by untrained individuals more difficult.

Under proper care, suffering can be alleviated and future episodes can be prevented. Once the disease is recognized, the stigma of the label "schizophrenia" can hinder the sufferer's ability to overcome the disease. As with any condition, the sufferer with schizophrenia is saddled with a medical diagnosis. There is no choice other than to accept it, to work with it, to be treated for it, and to understand it. In doing so, the sufferer is not defeated by it.

Mine is a 40-year success story. My hope is that this mental illness will be understood by society so that the stigma of the label "schizophrenia" will disappear and that those who suffer with the disease will be accepted and supported in their journey to wellness. It is also my hope that those afflicted with schizophrenia can, over time, return to wholly productive lives.

After beginning treatment for multiple myeloma in February 2018, I have gradually felt better. I now have energy and stamina, and my blood chemistries are normal. In a recent sermon given at my church, my minister reflected on healing in this way:

"We can be healed without a cure because Jesus heals and He is eternal."

God heals eternally to resurrect us. In this context, we can be healed from the affliction without a cure. We can live with the confidence of God's final triumph in Jesus' Resurrection.

## Thankfulness

In all that I have been through, I firmly believe a healthy attitude begins with gratitude, and gratitude is grounded in humble thankfulness. Thankfulness is a place to which you arrive after you have gone down all the wrong paths of your own desires, gotten lost or confused, become lonely or angry, and have found people willing to steer your spirit back toward the Holy with their love, compassion, hope, and grace. It is in this loving guidance that gratitude is born and blossoms. Some do it by the light of the Holy, others by their courage, and still others by their commitment to you. It is your thankfulness that allows you to see the gifts of their companionship.

Dr. Maloney gave me hope and helped restore me to relationship with others. He birthed my voice by his devoted listening, concern, and commitment to me. He opened to me a life humbled by my brokenness. He steered my spirit back to me. I spoke with him of the many things that troubled me and whenever I spoke of my understanding of God or Jesus, he would quietly point heavenward. I am deeply thankful for that.

## Resilience, Perseverance and Loyalty

Mary responds to the realities of life with resilience, perseverance, and loyalty. Always with a positive attitude, she loves when it is most difficult, helps when it is most needed, forgives the worst, and stands true when it is most necessary.

The pain of her experience with my illness has deepened her relationship with the Lord. She has been able to respond to others with love and forgiveness. The perseverance, learned from her mother, allows her to navigate through tough times. Able to bounce back from momentary difficulties great or small, she soldiers on with the life God has given her. She has always been responsible and accountable with her voice and her actions.

Mary is a people-person, always allowing others to shine around her. She is not one to be at the center of attention, but content to stand to the side in public situations. Well-meaning and forthright, her spoken words are well-taken from a sound mind, her own experience, and good old common sense.

Mary is a loyal, loving friend. Her graciousness and kindness to me throughout my illness have been a precious gift. Her steadfast love for me has been the healing balm that has, in large measure, allowed me to heal.

## Live Eternally

I remember how it was for me when I turned to Jesus after realizing I was suffering with mental illness. At the time, the outward manifestation of my life was unsettled and inwardly confused. In reflection, I was in the wilderness of my life. I was at a place in my life where nothing was working for me. Even after hearing about this Jesus, I was still wandering.

One day, I awoke and sensed that the time had arrived. For the first time in my life, I realized that I needed to repent. I knew I needed to knock at His door. After some consideration, I did so, asking forgiveness in a simple prayer.

After some time, I realized something was different. A flood of God's love came over me in the Spirit of this Jesus, and the door was open. I felt supported. I felt lighter and perceived a buoyancy of new joy. I felt that I was traveling with new spirit with someone protecting me. I felt carried. As I began to risk putting my burdens down, I picked up the Bible and felt I could rest in the arms of God's love. My sense of being, rushed by the world's ways, began to subside; I could take a deep breath in a moment of refreshment while reading God's word.

The love of God introduced me to His grace. I began to see the beauty of creation more clearly. My body reacted with the release from tension, anxiety, and fear. I felt quietly responsive to the creation around me. I started to think anew that God was with me, and I knew He was there to hear my prayer, to steady me, to comfort me.

I felt excited by the joy I had found. I started to speak from Jesus' perspective about the love of neighbor and the Father. The Holy Spirit gave me access to the Father's Kingdom—I felt His profound love. I knocked at His door and He answered as he said he would. Jesus now walks with me in a way that assures me He has my back. When I accepted Jesus, I realized God wiped out my transgressions. I could breathe, stand up straight, be honest, have courage, and love myself as I brought Jesus' spirit into my life.

Jesus loves me. He always has and always will. He wants to give me the life He has always wanted for me in the Father's plan. I am beginning to feel separate from the affairs of the world. I am new. I am effective. I have a voice. My life is beginning to work—all because of my willingness to repent and knock.

Jesus knew His time on the cross would be worth it. By his crucifixion and resurrection, I was forgiven and recreated. These are His gifts for me. My life is under the light of God's eternal providence.

I have decided to live eternally.

# God's Reassurance

*25 Therefore I say unto you, Take no thought for your life, what ye shall eat, or what ye shall drink; nor yet for your body, what ye shall put on. Is not the life more than meat, and the body than raiment?*

*26 Behold the fowls of the air: for they sow not, neither do they reap, nor gather into barns; yet your heavenly Father feedeth them. Are ye not much better than they?*

*27 Which of you by taking thought can add one cubit unto his stature?*

*28 And why take ye thought for raiment? Consider the lilies of the field, how they grow; they toil not, neither do they spin:*

*29 And yet I say unto you, That even Solomon in all his glory was not arrayed like one of these.*

*30 Wherefore, if God so clothe the grass of the field, which to-day is, and to-morrow is cast into the oven, shall he not much more clothe you, O ye of little faith?*

*31 Therefore take no thought, saying, What shall we eat?*

*or, What shall we drink? or, Wherewithal shall we be clothed?*

*32 (For after all these things do the Gentiles seek:) for your heavenly Father knoweth that ye have need of all these things.*

*33 But seek ye first the kingdom of God, and his righteousness; and all these things shall be added unto you.*

*34 Take therefore no thought for the morrow: for the morrow shall take thought for the things of itself. Sufficient unto the day is the evil thereof.*[14]

Matthew 6:25-34
King James Version

# Acknowledgments

FROM THE DEEPEST PART of my being, I would like to thank all the many family members and friends who were devastated and bewildered from day one, yet persevered with love and acceptance in their attempts to understand behavior, often strange, unbecoming, and out of place.

I thank my late parents who in their confrontation of the disease were sadly puzzled yet soldiered on, slow to criticize and admonish.

I am grateful for Andy's recognition of me as a loving brother, not just his twin. It has been life affirming. In our later years, we are closer than we have ever been.

I thank my sister Emily for her kindness and understanding throughout.

I would like to recognize my long-time friend Nolean Deskins, who never failed to show her love and support to me in the work environment. She remains a close friend after 35 years.

Also at the workplace, Carlos Lago, Allen Maples, and Jim Kent were sojourners with me and I remember them as the truest of friends.

I would like to thank Thomas Small, a security guard at EPA, who is also a minister, who took the time to listen. He encouraged me to rely on faith in the face of doubt.

Reverend Kathleen Moore championed me in my growth as a Christian and offered me the opportunity to become an Elder in my church. She was senior minister of First Christian Church of Falls Church (Disciples of Christ) at the time.

Lunette Arledge, music director at my church, and Thomas Beveridge, music director of the New Dominion Chorale and of the National Men's Chorus (until its close), were both instrumental in birthing my spoken and singing voices. They have offered me the sheer joy of singing in the Washington, D.C. metropolitan area.

Dr. John Maloney remains supremely skilled in medicine management and treatment plans for me, as well as being very patient with me in his listening. Together, we have tackled the challenge of a disability and confronted it. I have learned ways to live with the affliction under his tutelage and care.

I am grateful to Nick Ellyn, a good friend, who listened with knowledge, comfort, and compassion. It was with his encouragement and in his company that we first visited Greece.

I would be remiss without acknowledging my wife Mary and my brother Jim for their unrelenting and steadfast support. The recollections and the writing of this book have been a journey in itself.

All of these individuals have enriched my life and sustained my faith in my struggle. I am indebted to them all and thank them deeply for their supportive contribution to bringing me forward to full participation in life.

# Bibliography

Chalice Hymnal. Chalice Press. 1995.

Chambers, Oswald. *The Complete Works of Oswald Chambers.* Discovery House ® 2000. p. 1049.

Clemmer, Mary, Editor *Ballads for Little Folk: The Poems of Alice and Phoebe Cary.* Hurd and Houghton. 1874.

King James Version. American Bible Society. New York. 1611 (Public Domain).

Osler, William.

Rampersad, Arnold, Editor. *The Collected Poems of Langston Hughes.* Alfred A. Knopf/ Vintage. 1994.

# Author Bio

**Wendel Miser**

I grew up in the same home in New England with my brother Jim. I was, however, preoccupied with my twin brother, Andy, in our formative years and through high school. It was in high school that I met my wife, Mary, marrying her in September 1972, after finishing at Cornell College in Mt. Vernon, Iowa in June.

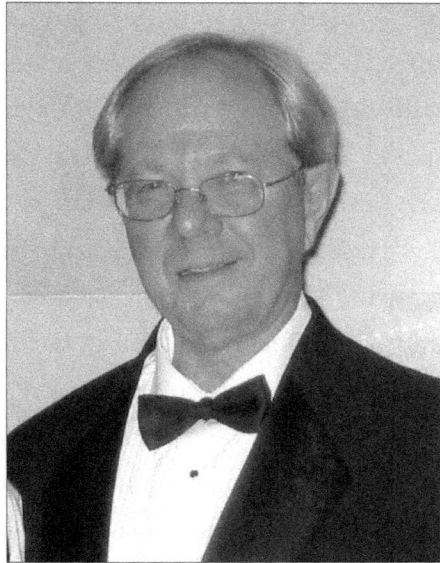

I received a Master of Science degree from the University of Illinois in 1975, after studying Zoology and Limnology. After graduate school, I worked with Mary's father in his painting business before accepting a position in the Office of Solid Waste at the United States Environmental Protection Agency in Washington, D.C. in 1977.

I began with their program of pesticide disposal for a short time and then became a project officer, managing the program side for the Agency's contract office. Working with the contract officer, I helped the staff with contract pre-award and post-award requirements for their work. In that capacity, I was involved for 23 years in the development of a nationwide hazardous waste management program. Subsequently, I moved to the Office's municipal waste program that was promoting recycling and sustainability programs at the time.

While not at work during the latter half of my career, I became interested in singing. For the better part of 20 years, I was involved with the New Dominion Chorale and the National Men's Chorus in the Washington, D.C. area. The New Dominion Chorale featured works by the Great Masters, while the National Men's Chorus showcased works specially arranged by the music director for the Chorus. Memorable concerts were given at the National Cathedral and the Kennedy Center as well as the National Gallery of Art, Washington, D.C. For six years, I served on the Board of Directors of the National Men's Chorus, assisting with grant activities.

I live with my wife in Arlington, Virginia with our two cats, Linus and Madeleine. We attend church regularly in Falls Church, Virginia. I have kept a faith-based journal for 38 years. In overcoming schizophrenia and finding joy, I have entered into full participation in life.

# Author Bio

**James S. Miser, MD**

I grew up on the East Coast of the United States with my father, mother, two younger twin brothers, and a younger sister, spending the majority of time in New England. My father was a mathematician with a PhD in this field, and he was an operations research and systems analysis professional. My mother had a Master of Science degree in Child Development; she spent most of our formative years caring for us as we grew and developed. We were a normal family and could not know what was to befall Wendel at the age of 28 years.

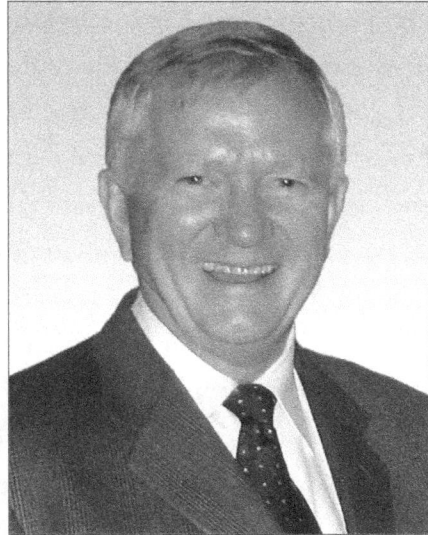

I am a Pediatric Hematologist and Oncologist and have taken care of children with cancer and blood diseases for almost 50 years. I received a Bachelor of Arts degree from Dartmouth College, Hanover, New Hampshire, in 1969, majoring in Religion. While there I also was the director of the college's acapella singing group.

In the summers during high school and college, I taught tennis to children. Although I intended to be a mathematician, I decided to spend my life working with children and entered Dartmouth Medical School with the intention to be a pediatrician. I subsequently transferred to the University of Washington, Seattle, Washington where I received a Doctor of Medicine in 1973 and trained in Pediatrics and Pediatric Hematology and Oncology.

At the beginning of my experience caring for children with cancer, I accepted the Lord Jesus Christ as Lord and Savior of my life. This has been an important relationship for me since that time. I have worked as a Pediatric Hematologist/Oncologist at Ohio State University, the National Institutes of Health, Mayo Clinic, the University of Washington, where I was granted the position of Professor of Pediatrics, and City of Hope National Medical Center, where I was Chairman of Pediatrics. I also served as President and Chief Medical Officer at City of Hope National Medical Center as it developed a comprehensive cancer center.

I have authored more than 100 manuscripts and book chapters. I worked as medical director and served as Chairman of the American Board of Directors of a child rescue organization— Christian Salvation Service, in Taipei, Taiwan, serving children and women. During this time, I was also Chair Professor of Pediatrics at Taipei Medical University where I was challenged to develop a Pediatric Hematology/Oncology program for the University.

I also served as Chairman of the Board of Directors of a Christian High School in southern California and currently serve as Chairman of the Board of Directors of a nonprofit organization supporting children with cancer and their families.

My wife Angela and I have adopted 10 children, many with significant challenges. I live in Wales with my wife and five of the children. I enjoy walking, reading, playing tennis, and singing. I attend church with my wife in the Church of Wales. The mission of my life has been to serve children, both personally and professionally, especially those with significant challenges in their lives.

I have been close to my brother, Wendel, in his journey with schizophrenia and shared the initial horror, the subsequent anxiety of the ups and downs of his experience, and now the joy of his overcoming. It has been a privilege to travel his journey and to write this book with him.

# Endnotes

1    Luke 17:11-19 AV.

2    Rom. 8:38-39 AV.

3    Edwin Markham, Chalice Hymnal (Missouri: Chalice Press, 1995).

4    Luke 2:8-14 AV.

5    Langston Hughes, "Dreams," in The Collected Poems of Langston Hughes, ed. Arnold Rampersad (New York: Alfred A. Knopf/Vintage, 1994).

6    Ezek. 36:24-28 AV.

7    Rom. 8:38-39 AV.

8    Deut. 8:3 AV.

9    John 14:27 AV.

10   Isa. 49:16 AV.

11   Alice Cary and Phoebe Cary, Ballads for Little Folk: The Poems of Alice and Phoebe Cary, ed. Mary Clemmer (New York: Hurd and Houghton, 1874).

12   Phil. 4:6-7 AV.

13   Matt. 17:20 AV.

14   Matt. 17:20 AV.

www.ingramcontent.com/pod-product-compliance
Lightning Source LLC
Chambersburg PA
CBHW032058020426
42335CB00011B/400